CASE REVIEW
Breast Imaging

Series Editor
David M. Yousem, MD, MBA
Professor of Radiology
Director of Neuroradiology
Russell H. Morgan Department of Radiology and Radiological Science
The Johns Hopkins Medical Institutions
Baltimore, Maryland

Other Volumes in the CASE REVIEW Series
Brain Imaging
Cardiac Imaging
Gastrointestinal Imaging
General and Vascular Ultrasound
Genitourinary Imaging
Head and Neck Imaging
Musculoskeletal Imaging
Nuclear Medicine
Obstetric and Gynecologic Ultrasound
Pediatric Imaging
Spine Imaging
Thoracic Imaging
Vascular and Interventional Imaging

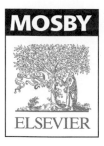

Emily F. Conant, MD
Professor of Radiology
Chief, Breast Imaging
University of Pennsylvania Medical Center
Philadelphia, Pennsylvania

Cecilia M. Brennecke, MD
Medical Director
Director of Breast Imaging
Johns Hopkins at Green Spring
Baltimore, Maryland

CASE REVIEW

Breast Imaging

CASE REVIEW SERIES

MOSBY
ELSEVIER

1600 John F. Kennedy Blvd.
Suite 1800
Philadelphia, PA 19103-2899

BREAST IMAGING: CASE REVIEW
Copyright © 2006 by Mosby, Inc., an affiliate of Elsevier Inc.

ISBN-13: 978-0-323-01746-6
ISBN-10: 0-323-01746-0

NOTICE

ISBN-13: 978-0-323-01746-6
ISBN-10: 0-323-01746-0

Acquisitions Editor: Meghan McAteer
Editorial Assistants: Elizabeth Schweizer; Ryan Creed
Marketing Manager: Emily Christie

Printed in the United States of America.

Last digit is the print number: 9 8 7 6 5 4 3

To all the patients who continue to teach me about how important caring is.
EFC

To the team at Green Spring Station, and to Mark, Ben and Eli, the men who make it possible.
CMB

My experience in teaching medical students, residents, fellows, practicing radiologists, and clinicians has been that they love the case conference format more than any other approach. I hope that the reason for this is not a reflection on my lecturing ability, but rather that people stay awake, alert, and on their toes more when they are in the hot seat (or may be the next person to assume the hot seat). In the dozens of continuing medical education courses I have directed, the case review sessions are almost always the most popular parts of the courses.

The idea of this Case Review series grew out of a need for books designed as exam preparation tools for the resident, fellow, or practicing radiologist about to take the boards or the certificate of additional qualification (CAQ) exams. Anxiety runs extremely high concerning the content of these exams, administered as unknown cases. Residents, fellows, and practicing radiologists are very hungry for formats that mimic this exam setting and that cover the types of cases they will encounter and have to accurately describe. In addition, books of this ilk serve as excellent practical reviews of a field and can help a practicing board-certified radiologist keep his or her skills sharpened. Thus heads banged together, and Mosby and I arrived at the format of the volume herein, which is applied consistently to each volume in the series. We believe that these volumes will strengthen the ability of the reader to interpret studies. By formatting the individual cases so that they can "stand alone," these case review books can be read in a leisurely fashion, a case at a time, on the whim of the reader.

The content of each volume is organized into three sections based on difficulty of interpretation and/or the rarity of the lesion presented. There are the Opening Round cases, which graduating radiology residents should have relatively little difficulty mastering. The Fair Game section consists of cases that require more study, but most people should get into the ballpark with their differential diagnoses. Finally, there is the Challenge section. Most fellows or fellowship-trained practicing radiologists will be able to mention entities in the differential diagnoses of these challenging cases, but one shouldn't expect to consistently "hit home runs" à la Mark McGwire. The Challenge cases are really designed to whet one's appetite for further reading on these entities and to test one's wits. Within each of these sections, the selection of cases is entirely random, as one would expect at the boards (in your office or in Louisville).

For many cases in this series, a specific diagnosis may not be what is expected—the quality of the differential diagnosis and the inclusion of appropriate options are most important. Teaching how to distinguish between the diagnostic options (taught in the question and answer and comment sections) will be the goal of the authors of each Case Review volume.

The best way to go through these books is to look at the images, guess the diagnosis, answer the questions, and then turn the page for the answers. If there are two cases on a page, do them two at a time. No peeking!

Mosby (through the strong work of Liz Corra) and I have recruited most of the authors of THE REQUISITES series (editor, James Thrall, MD) to create Case Review books for their subspecialties. To meet the needs of certain subspecialties and to keep each of the volumes to a consistent, practical size, some specialties will have more than one volume (e.g., ultrasound, interventional and vascular radiology, and neuroradiology). Nonetheless, the pleasing tone of THE REQUISITES series and its emphasis on condensing the fields of radiology into its foundations will be inculcated into the Case Review volumes. In many situations, THE REQUISITES authors have enlisted new coauthors to breathe a novel approach and excitement into the cases submitted. I think the fact that so many of THE REQUISITES authors are "on board" for this new series is a testament to their dedication to teaching. I hope that the success of THE REQUISITES is duplicated with the new Case Review series. Just as THE REQUISITES series provides coverage of the essentials in each sub-specialty and successfully meets that overwhelming need in the market, I hope that the Case Review series successfully meets the overwhelming need in the market for practical, focused case reviews.

David M. Yousem, MD, MBA

Breast imaging has grown from the early modality of xerographic or plain film mammography to a thriving, bustling diagnostic practice that includes the use of ultrasound, nuclear medicine, PET imaging, and MRI. Interventional procedures now dominate the breast imager's time as well, affording greater clinical interaction with the patient. The field continues to be a vibrant source of innovative techniques as radiologists hope to stem the tide of breast cancer in the world.

In selecting authors for this edition I listened to my wife, who swears by her doctor, Peggy Brennecke, as the consummate breast imager: intelligent, caring, and thorough. Dr. Brennecke is joined by one of my former colleagues from the University of Pennsylvania, Emily Conant, who combines these same compassionate traits with an active academic practice and a research-oriented mind. Together Drs. Conant and Brennecke have forged an outstanding new edition of the Case Review Series, with a wonderful collection of breast imaging cases that I believe will be instructive to all.

The philosophy of the Case Review Series is to review each specialty in a challenging, interactive way. Each book in the series has gradations of difficulty so that the reader can assess his or her proficiency and can use this self-evaluation to guide continued education. Because each case in the book is distinct, this is the kind of text that can be picked up and read at any time in your day, in your career.

I am very pleased to welcome the *Breast Imaging: Case Review* edition to the ever-growing Case Review family, which includes *Cardiac Imaging* by Gautham Reddy and Robert Steiner; *Vascular and Interventional Imaging* by Suresh Vedantham and Jennifer Gould; *Pediatric Imaging* by Rob Ward and Hans Blickman; *Nuclear Medicine* by Harvey A. Zeissman and Patrician Rehm; *General and Vascular Ultrasound* by William D. Middleton; *Musculoskeletal Imaging* by Joseph Yu; *Obstetric and Gynecologic Ultrasound* by Al Kurtz and Pam Johnson; *Spine Imaging* by Brian Bowen; *Thoracic Imaging* by Phil Boiselle and Theresa McLoud; *Genitourinary Imaging* by Ron Zagoria, William Mayo-Smith, and Glenn Tung; *Gastrointestinal Imaging* by Peter Feczko and Robert Halpert; *Brain Imaging* by Laurie Loevner; and *Head and Neck Imaging* by David M. Yousem and Ana Carolina B. S. da Motta.

David M. Yousem, MD, MBA

Breast imaging is endlessly challenging. It is also endlessly humbling and endlessly rewarding. The feeling one gets on finding an early cancer, especially when it is a subtle finding, is a mixture of accomplishment and regret. On the one hand, it is exciting to find the cancer at its earliest stage. On the other hand, the patient has been handed a diagnosis that changes her life.

Breast imagers get involved in the care of their patients. They talk to the patient, examine the patient, recommend the next imaging step, perform biopsies, perform ultrasound. They make decisions about management. In every mammography report, the radiologist maps out a diagnosis and a treatment plan.

Breast imagers are held to a high standard. We track our misses, our false positives and false negatives, as well as our successes. We have a responsibility to ourselves, to our patients, even to the federal government, to perform to the highest standards in order to find the cancer at its earliest stage.

This is a book that takes you through the many facets of breast imaging. It is intended to illustrate a variety of imaging tools and to offer thoughts on management of many breast conditions. We hope you will find the information useful, and at the end feel more confident in your ability to search for and find breast cancer.

Emily F. Conant, MD
Cecilia M. Brennecke, MD

I've known Dave Yousem a long time; we were residents together at Johns Hopkins Hospital 20 years ago. When he asked me to write this book, I refused. I guess you can see who won the day; here is the book. Dave is one of the most energetic, optimistic, not to mention smartest people I know.

I depend daily on the expertise, generosity, and friendship of Dr. Wendie Berg. I am fortunate to share the practice with her. I owe a large debt of gratitude to Nagi Khouri, as well as to Lisa Mullen, Bruce Copeland, and Susan Harvey. My research assistant, Cindy Neorr, helps me immeasurably. I wouldn't have images to show you without the talents of the mammography technical staff, led by Stephanie Jackson, and all the staff at Johns Hopkins/American Radiology Services at Green Spring Station.

My coauthor, Emily Conant, is a very smart academic breast specialist, the perfect complement to my clinical experience. I thank her particularly for her attention to detail, so important in the practice of radiology and the writing of a book. Many thanks also to Meghan McAteer at Elsevier and to Peggy Gordon.

My family bore the brunt of the book. My husband, Mark Hyman, covered for me during all the times we needed at least one parent around. Without him, I would not be writing this page. Our sons, Ben and Eli, continue to inspire, critique, and humble me. Thanks, most of all, to you three.

Cecilia M. Brennecke, MD

Like my coauthor Peggy, when Dave Yousem called and asked if I was interested in writing this book, I said. "No way." He called again and I said, "No thanks." About a year later he called again, and I finally said, "Maybe. . . ." Finally I agreed. In agreeing to coauthor this book, my main goal was to convert my old analog teaching file (the messy pile of old films that was in my office) into a digital directory of breast imaging cases (the hard drive now attached to this computer). The book part seemed like a bonus! But now seeing this case review complete, I find myself extremely satisfied with the result, and I would like to thank Dave for being so persistent. Dave, you have a great team working on the book, particularly Meghan McAteer at Elsevier and Peggy Gordon at P.M. Gordon Associates. It has been a pleasure to work with both of them, and I thank them both for their hard work.

Peggy Brennecke—I have learned so much from the cases and insights that you brought to this book. Thank you for being such a wonderfully patient partner, and thank goodness we live only a train ride away! Maybe in a few years we can do this again!

A special thanks goes to Rose DiCicco, who listened intently and transcribed all my dictated tapes of cases. You are amazing and I could not have done any of this without you. Plus you keep me sane on a daily basis here in our little corner at the University of Pennsylvania. We are a great team.

My family has also been intimately involved in the production of this book. From the beginning, my husband Jon and our kids, Hannah, Alice, and Sam, have all thought that it was really neat that I was trying to write a book. Over the past year they have shared the kitchen table, the top of my bed, and the living room floor with the spread of images and pages of questions. Despite the mess, they have understood and given me space and time and I thank them. I know they think it is even neater that the book has finally been published!

In looking back over the short 17 years of my career, I have been extremely lucky to have had the amazing mentorship of Rosalind Troupin, Igor Laufer, and Wally Miller. Early in my career these three amazing radiologists introduced me to the intrigue of image interpretation and the challenge of teaching. Because of their infectious enthusiasm for teaching, I can't imagine myself in any other career than that of academic radiology. It is a great honor to have been trained by you, to work with you, and to be continually inspired by you.

I must also acknowledge all the residents with whom I have been fortunate enough to read a case. They continue to question and challenge me, forcing me to think and teach in new ways. To paraphrase Wally Miller, "The greatest reward in teaching is to see one's students go out to teach others." Daily we teach the residents and fellows and daily they learn from both our good and better practices to hopefully become better than we are. That is my greatest reward: to see our students take joy in teaching others to improve on what we do today.

Finally, I would like to thank both of my loving parents for supporting me in my quests over the years—whether it was to be a ski bum, an artist, a traveler, a doctor, a teacher, a writer (?), and, most importantly, a wife and mother. You are wonderful role models, and I hope that I will continue to enjoy the balance in life that you have provided for me and seem to continue to find with each other.

Emily F. Conant, MD

Opening Round

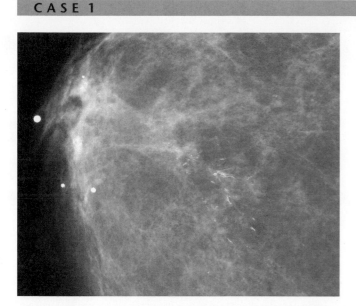

A 40-year-old woman presents for a baseline screening mammogram. A magnification view in the CC projection demonstrates microcalcifications of DCIS.

1. What population makes up a screening population?

2. What population makes up a diagnostic population?

3. What is prevalence screening, and what is the approximate cancer detection rate in this population?

4. What is incidence screening, and what is the approximate cancer detection rate in this population?

Incidence and Prevalence

1. Screening patients are asymptomatic patients without any signs or symptoms of breast cancer.

2. Diagnostic patients are "problem-solving" patients who present with symptoms or signs of possible breast cancer. Diagnostic patients are also patients who are called back from screening for additional imaging of a screen-detected abnormality.

3. Prevalence screening is first-round screening where no prior films were available. The cancer detection rate is 6–10 per 1000.

4. Incidence screening is the repeated attendance to screening programs. The cancer detection rate is lower, approximately 2–4 per 1000.

Reference

Bassett LW, Jackson VP, Jahan R, Fu YS, Gold RH: *Diagnosis of Diseases of the Breast*, Philadelphia, 1997, Saunders.

Cross-Reference

Ikeda, *Breast Imaging: THE REQUISITES*, p 37.

Comment

Screening mammography refers to the routine imaging of patients who have no signs or symptoms of breast cancer. Screening is generally recommended yearly for all women 40 years of age and older. The initiation of routine screening may begin earlier in some high-risk women. Screening studies are often read in "batches" in high-volume breast centers, and if a lesion or questionable abnormality is detected, the patient is called back on another day for a diagnostic mammographic study and often for ultrasound. Therefore, diagnostic patients are those women who have signs or symptoms of breast cancer either on screening studies ("callbacks") or on breast exam (lump, thickening, nipple discharge, etc.). These diagnostic studies are read while the patient is in the breast center so that the study may be tailored to the patient's needs. Frequently, diagnostic mammographic studies use additional nonroutine images, such as 90° lateral views, spot compression, and/or magnification views. A radiologist is on site, overseeing the imaging of the diagnostic patient.

The rate of screen-detected cancers varies depending on the population screened. In an average-risk population that has never had a prior mammogram, the average detection rate or "prevalence" of cancer is approximately 6–10 cancers detected per 1000 patients. The cancer rate in this previously unscreened population is higher than in a population that has been undergoing routine screening. The "incidence" of cancer in a population refers to the number of new cancers detected each year not present previously (or at least not mammographically detectable). The incidence of breast cancer is approximately 2–4 cases per 1000. In other words, the term *prevalence* refers to the estimated number of people who have breast cancer at any given time, and the term *incidence* refers to the number of new cases diagnosed each year.

Notes

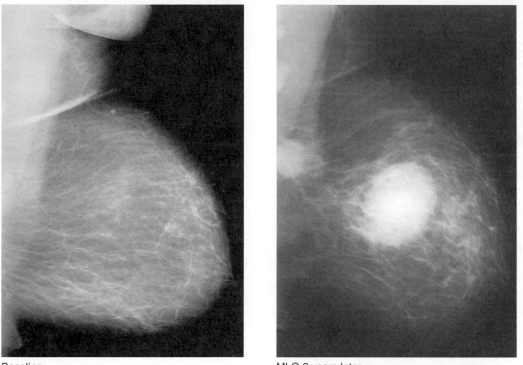

Baseline   MLO 3 years later

1. This 43-year-old woman had a baseline study (left) and presented 3 years later with a palpable right mass (right). What secondary signs of breast cancer are seen in this case?

2. What are the American Cancer Society (ACS) and the American College of Radiology (ACR) screening guidelines for women 40 years and older?

3. What is the reported reduction of breast cancer mortality associated with routine screening?

4. What is the incidence of breast cancer for women in the United States?

Screening Guidelines

1. There is a large high-density mass with surrounding edema and skin thickening. There are also several enlarged nodes seen in the axilla.

2. The ACS and ACR recommend yearly mammographic screening for all women age 40 years or older.

3. 20–40% reduction with routine screening.

4. One in eight women will develop breast cancer in her lifetime.

References

American Cancer Society Web site: www.cancer.org.

Bassett LW, Jackson VP, Jahan R, Fu YS, Gold RH: *Diagnosis of Diseases of the Breast*, Philadelphia, 1997, Saunders.

Cross-Reference

Ikeda, *Breast Imaging: THE REQUISITES*, p 1.

Comment

The goal of screening mammography is to detect breast cancers as early as possible, before they become palpable and have associated signs of advanced disease. Early detection provides a better prognosis and allows women more treatment options. American women on average, have a 1 in 8 lifetime risk for developing breast cancer. The chance of dying from breast cancer is approximately 1 in 33. The ACS estimates that in 2004 there were 211,240 women diagnosed with breast cancer and 40,410 breast cancer–related deaths. This estimate of the death rate represents a decrease compared to previous years and is attributed to earlier detection and more effective treatments.

Randomized controlled trials of breast cancer screening with mammography have reportedly decreased the breast cancer mortality rate by 20–40%. In 1997, following a consensus conference that reviewed the cumulative data of all the randomized controlled screening trials, the ACS issued guidelines recommending that all woman undergo annual screening mammography beginning at the age of 40 years. The ACS also recommends that beginning at age 20, every woman should practice monthly breast exams and have a clinical breast exam by a health care provider at least every 3 years.

Notes

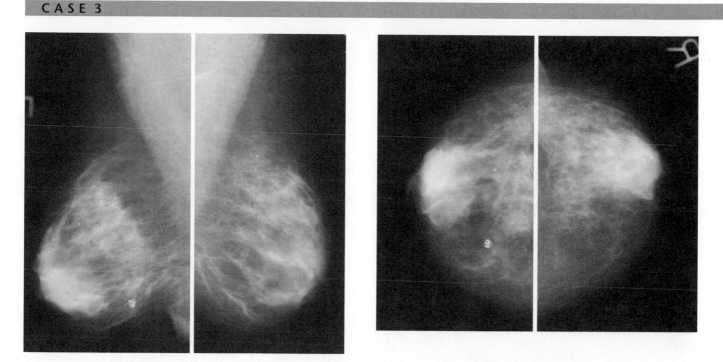

1. What are some risk factors for developing an invasive breast cancer?

2. How does estrogen play a role in breast cancer risk?

3. What percentage of breast cancers are related to known genetic mutations?

4. How does the history of prior breast biopsies impact personal risk for developing an invasive breast carcinoma?

Risk Factors

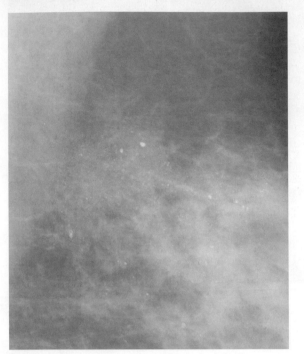

Benign regional punctate calcifications of adenosis

1. Increasing age, a personal history of prior breast cancer or high-risk lesion on breast biopsy, a first-degree relative with breast cancer, and early menarche and late menopause are all associated with an increase risk of developing an invasive breast carcinoma.

2. Many years of unopposed estrogens are known to increase a woman's risk for breast cancer. This is evident in women who have never been pregnant and have early menarche and late menopause.

3. Less than 25% of breast cancers diagnosed are due to known genetic mutations. Therefore, the majority of breast cancers have no known genetic etiology.

4. The history of having had prior breast biopsies actually increases an individual's personal risk. The risk is proportional to the level of atypia seen on the breast biopsy, with a higher risk associated with histories of biopsies yielding ALH and ADH.

Reference
Bassett LW, Jackson VP, Jahan R, Fu YS, Gold RH: *Diagnosis of Diseases of the Breast*, Philadelphia, 1997, Saunders, p 308.

Cross-Reference
Ikeda, *Breast Imaging: THE REQUISITES*, p 25.

Comment

The majority of women diagnosed with breast cancer have no known risk factor other than their gender. Although there are many factors that appear to contribute to an individual's risk for breast cancer, only a few factors are considered significant. These include increasing age; a personal history of breast cancer or a prior biopsy yielding a high-risk lesion; and various genetic mutations, including BRCA1 and BRCA2. However, patients with known genetic mutations make up only a small percentage (<25%) of the number of women diagnosed with breast cancer. In many families considered to be at high risk due to multiple cancer histories, no known mutation has been found. Presumably, there are many other, unidentified genetic susceptibilities.

Prolonged levels of unopposed endogenous and exogenous estrogens are also thought to contribute to an elevated risk. For example, early menarche, late menopause, nulliparity and late age at first pregnancy, and, recently, prolonged use of HRT are all considered factors in the etiology of breast cancer, but the exact mechanism is not well understood.

A woman's history of prior breast biopsies is also helpful in defining her individual risk since there are quite a few benign yet atypical lesions of the breast that confer a higher risk of developing an invasive breast carcinoma. In particular, the category of epithelial proliferative changes, associated with atypia of either the ductal or the lobular type, has histologic features that are similar to those of carcinomas *in situ*. Retrospective studies have shown that women with prior biopsies yielding these atypical histologies (ADH and ALH) have a risk four or five times higher than that of women without these proliferative changes.

Notes

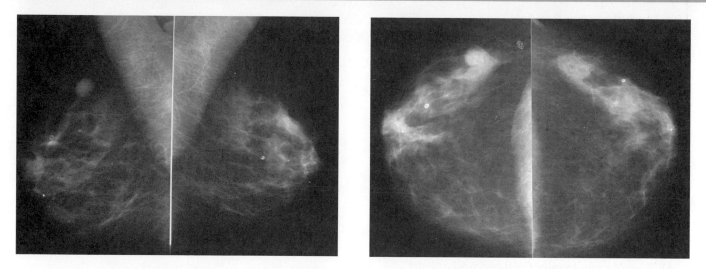

1. This patient presents for her annual mammogram. The round mass in the left upper outer breast has been shown to be a simple cyst. What is the breast density? What BI-RADS category would you give?

2. Are there standards for writing a mammogram report?

3. Why is standardization important?

4. What is the name of the federal law that mammography is governed by?

The Mammogram Report

1. There are scattered fibroglandular densities. There is a stable well-defined oval mass in the left upper outer breast, unchanged compared to prior exam. BI-RADS 2.

2. Yes, there are standards for reporting. The mammogram report should state the reason for the exam, the breast composition (or tissue density), description of the findings, comparison to previous exam, and the summary impression with BI-RADS code 0–6.

3. Standardization helps the patient and the referring physician know your exact interpretation of the mammogram. It provides concise, consistent reporting.

4. MQSA—Mammography Quality Standards Act.

Reference

American College of Radiology Breast Imaging Reporting and Data System, Reston, VA, 2003.

Cross-Reference

Ikeda, *Breast Imaging: THE REQUISITES*, p 37.

Comment

The mammogram report should follow a standard format, which includes the following elements:
1. Reason for exam—screening (routine) versus diagnostic (problem solving)
2. Tissue density (breast composition)
   a. Almost entirely fat (<25% glandular)
   b. Scattered fibroglandular densities (25–50% glandular)
   c. Heterogeneous dense, which could obscure detection of small masses (50–75% glandular)
   d. Extremely dense, which may lower the sensitivity of mammography (>75% glandular)
3. Description of any significant findings
   a. Mass
   b. Calcifications
   c. Architectural distortion
4. Comparison to previous exam, if available
5. Impression—include BI-RADS categories
   a. BI-RADS 1—negative
   b. BI-RADS 2—benign finding(s)
   c. BI-RADS 3—probably benign (<2% chance of malignancy)
   d. BI-RADS 4—suspicious abnormality, biopsy should be considered
   e. BI-RADS 5—highly suspicious, appropriate action should be taken (>95% chance of malignancy)
   f. BI-RADS 6—biopsy-proven cancer
   g. BI-RADS 0—incomplete, needs additional evaluation

The inclusion of a recommendation at the end of the report is good medical practice. This should state if the patient is to have her next mammogram at the standard interval, a follow-up at a short interval, or biopsy.

Screening mammography results should be limited to normal (BI-RADS 1 or 2) or incomplete (BI-RADS 0), needs more evaluation. Rarely is a BI-RADS 4 or 5 given at screening. Suspicious findings should be further evaluated with additional views prior to rendering a final impression. BI-RADS 3 is used after the full evaluation has been performed and the finding has a small chance of malignancy (<2%), and a short interval follow-up is recommended.

Notes

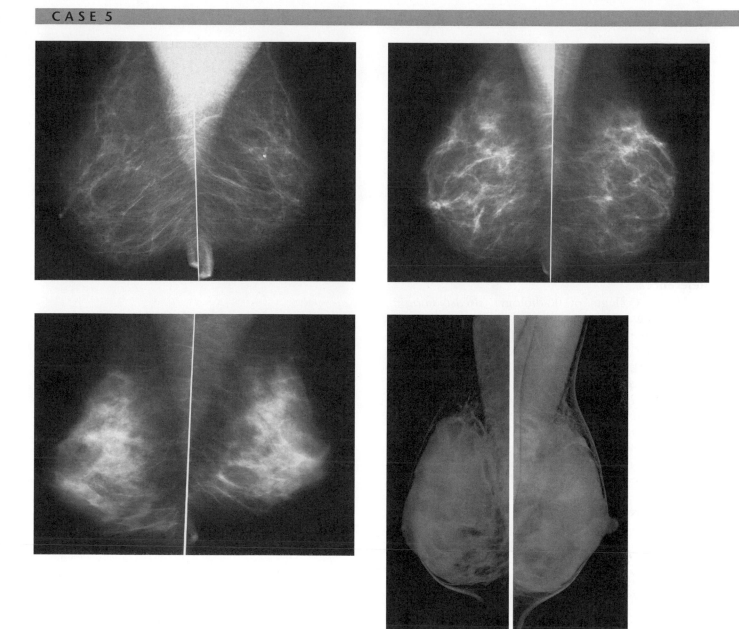

1. What are the differences between these four different patients?
2. Is it important to mention the tissue density in the mammogram report?
3. How does the breast density affect the ability to detect breast cancer?
4. Can breast density change with time or from other factors?

Breast Tissue Density Examples

1. These are all normal patients, who differ in tissue density.

2. It is important to give the tissue density because it gives the degree of confidence in excluding cancer.

3. Because the density of cancer is higher than that of fat, but similar to that of gland tissue, there is a greater ability to detect cancer when the tissue density contains more fat.

4. Breast density can change with pregnancy, lactation, advancing age, weight gain or loss, and disease states such as inflammation and malignancy.

References

American College of Radiology: *Breast Imaging Reporting and Data System (BI-RADS)*, Reston, VA, 2003, American College of Radiology.

Kerlikowske K, Carney PA, Geller B, Mandelson MT, Taplin SH, Malvin K, Ernster V, Urban N, Cutter G, Rosenberg R, Ballard-Barbash R: Performance of screening mammography among women with and without a first-degree relative with breast cancer, *Ann Intern Med* 133:855–863, 2000.

Lautin EM, Berlin L: Writing, signing, and reading the radiology report: Who is responsible and when? *Am J Roentgenol* 177:246–248, 2001.

Cross-Reference

Ikeda, *Breast Imaging: THE REQUISITES*, p 28.

Comment

Mammographic density is reported because it tells the referring physician the sensitivity of the mammogram in detecting breast cancer. In the fatty breast, the contrast between the background dark fat and the white tumor is the greatest; therefore, sensitivity for detecting cancer is the highest in this type of breast. In the dense breast, the background density is white, similar to the density of tumor, so a tumor can be missed.

The four-category system of breast density is as follows:

1. Almost entirely fat, <25% glandular

2. Scattered fibroglandular densities, 25–50% glandular

3. Heterogeneously dense, 50–75% glandular

4. Extremely dense, >75% glandular

Dense breasts are seen commonly in the young woman, and the density may decrease with age. The sensitivity of the mammogram varies with patient age and with breast density.

Notes

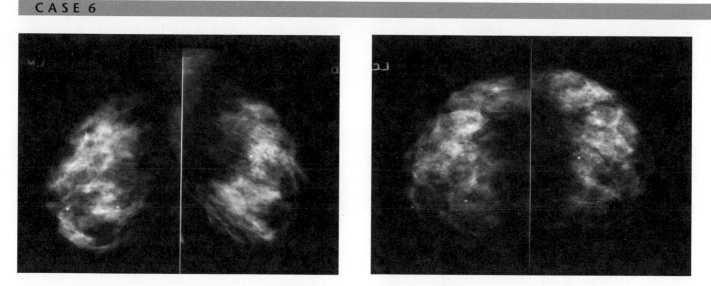

1. What is the breast density on the mammogram of this 82-year-old woman?

2. Does this breast tissue type indicate a higher risk of malignancy?

3. Is this tissue type more often seen in the premenopausal or postmenopausal patient?

4. In the postmenopausal woman, is this density more likely to be seen with hormone replacement therapy?

Case of Dense Breast in an 82-Year-Old

1. The tissue density is heterogeneously dense, 50% to 75% glandular.

2. Dense breasts have been shown in some studies to have an increased risk of breast cancer—four to six times the rate of less dense breasts.

3. This breast density is found more often in premenopausal women.

4. This breast density is more likely seen HRT, which causes increased generalized density on mammogram.

References

Harvey JA, Bovbjerg VE: Quantitative assessment of mammographic breast density: Relationship with breast cancer risk, *Radiology* 230:29–41, 2004.

Stomper PC, D'Souza DJ, DiNitto PA, Arredondo MA: Analysis of parenchymal density on mammograms in 1353 women 25–79 years old, *Am J Roentgenol* 167: 1261, 1996.

Cross-Reference

Ikeda, *Breast Imaging: THE REQUISITES*, p 28.

Comment

Denser breasts are commonly seen in mammography. This type of mammogram is more difficult to interpret because the radiographic density of the glandular tissue and a mass or cyst is similar, meaning that masses may be obscured in a dense breast. The dense tissue on the mammogram represents the ducts and lobules and also fibrous connective tissue. In a dense breast, there is relatively little fat interspersed between the glandular elements.

The increased density imparted an increased risk of breast cancer in several studies using a quantitative measurement of breast density, with an odds ratio of 4.0 or greater, meaning that women with dense breasts had a fourfold increase in risk of breast cancer compared to those with the least dense breasts. Due to the breast density and advanced age, older women with dense breasts may have a increased risk.

Breast tissue is responsive to hormone changes. Estrogen levels are higher in younger women, and after menopause, estrogen levels diminish and cause the breast lobules to regress. The mammogram then becomes less dense. Sixty-five percent of women in their twenties have at least 50% breast density. This decreases to 50% of women in their forties and to 30% of women in their seventies.

Hormone replacement therapy increases the glandular density of the breast in up to 73% of women, and the greatest increase in density occurs in the first year of use.

The 82-year-old patient reported here is not on hormone replacement therapy, and the mammogram is unchanged compared to previous exams.

Notes

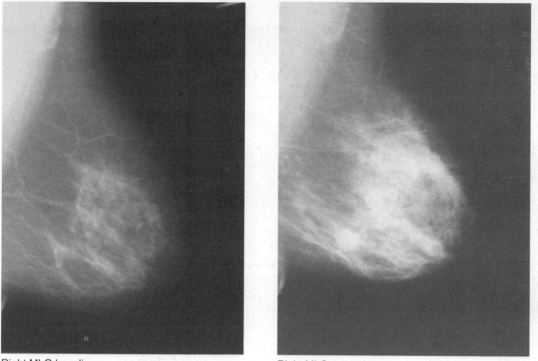

Right MLO baseline   Right MLO 1 year later

1. The patient presents with bilateral breast tenderness and an increase in the size of the breasts. (Images from only the right are shown, but the change was symmetric bilaterally.) There are no focal findings on breast exam. Describe the change over time in the breast density.

2. What pertinent clinical questions should be asked of the patient?

3. Is ultrasound indicated in this patient?

4. Discuss management of the clinical situation and the appropriate final BI-RADS category.

Hormone Replacement Therapy

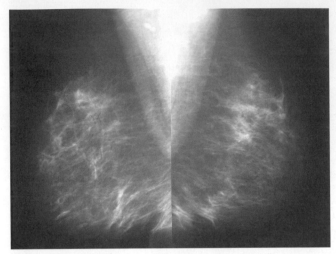

MLO, premenopausal

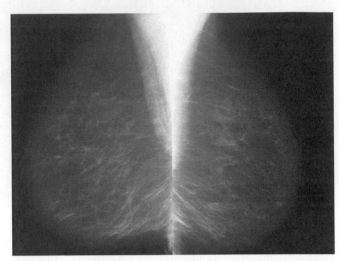

MLO, postmenopausal

1. The right breast image shows an increase in density and size. Previously, the breasts had scattered fibroglandular densities, and now they are heterogeneously dense.

2. The patient should be questioned regarding any exogenous hormonal therapy.

3. Ultrasound is not indicated unless there is a focal area of palpable concern.

4. Routine follow-up is recommended; BI-RADS category 2: benign.

References

Berkowitz JE, Gatewood OM, Goldblum LE, Gayler BW: Hormonal replacement therapy: Mammographic manifestations, *Radiology* 174:199–201, 1990.

Rutter CM, Mandelson MT, Laya MB, Taplin S: Changes in breast density associated with initiation, discontinuation, and continuing use of hormone replacement therapy, *J Am Med Assoc* 285(2):171–176, 2001.

Stomper PC, Van Voorhis BJ, Ravnikar VA, Meyer JE: Mammographic changes associated with postmenopausal hormone replacement therapy: A longitudinal study, *Radiology* 174:487–490, 1990.

Cross-Reference

Ikeda, *Breast Imaging: THE REQUISTIES*, p 302.

Comment

The breasts bilaterally show an increase in density. They are now considered heterogeneously dense, whereas before they had scattered fibroglandular densities. The most common cause of bilaterally symmetric increasing density that involves the glandular tissue and not the skin (no edema or skin thickening) is exogenous hormonal therapy, as in this case. The patient had begun taking a combined estrogen and progesterone supplement.

Normally, as a woman enters menopause, there are involutional changes that occur in the breast parenchyma. The volume of the mammographically dense areas tends to decrease as the glandular elements involute (as in the case on this page). HRT reverses the normal involution, and histologically the breast epithelium and stromal elements proliferate. This is due to the effects of the estrogen component of the HRT. The progesterone effects include an increase in epithelial mytotic activity and lobular hyperplasia. Women on HRT may experience breast pain. This occurs in approximately 25% of women and appears to be dose dependent.

The imaging evaluation must be based on the clinical findings. Ultrasound is not indicated when there is a diffused bilateral increase in density when it can be explained by exogenous hormonal therapy. In our practice, we do not generally perform ultrasound on women who have bilateral diffuse breast pain. If there is a focal area of tenderness or an area of palpable concern, a directed ultrasound is performed. In cases such as this one, it is not necessary to terminate the HRT but, rather, routine follow-up is recommended. Occasionally, the mammographic and clinical findings may be more unilateral and focal, in which case physical exam, directed ultrasound, and possibly MRI may be needed to exclude a developing malignancy.

Notes

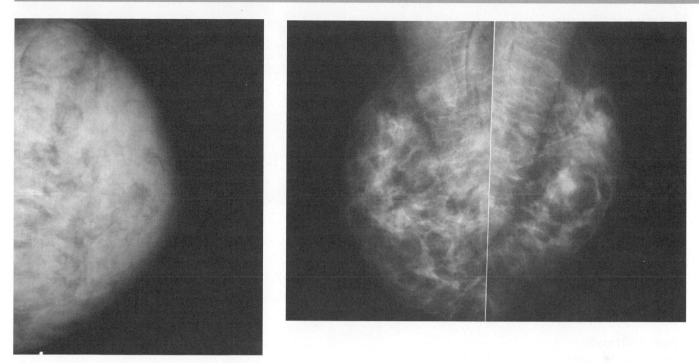

1. Describe the difference between the two mammograms of the same patient taken four years apart.

2. What condition could explain the change?

3. Why is screening mammography not routinely performed during lactation?

4. The patient presented with a palpable lump while lactating. Is mammography indicated?

Lactational Change

1. The gland tissue initially is extremely dense. The same patient four years later has heterogeneously dense breasts.

2. Lactation.

3. The density of the breast tissue during lactation lowers the sensitivity of the exam.

4. Mammography is indicated in the evaluation of a lump. Palpable cancer may present as microcalcifications, which may only be seen on mammography. However, ultrasound should also be performed.

Reference

Ahn BY, Kim HH, Moon WK, Pisano ED, Kim HS, Cha ES, Kim JS, Oh KK, Park SH: Pregnancy- and lactation-associated breast cancer: Mammographic and sonographic findings, *J Ultrasound Med* 22:491, 2003.

Cross-Reference

Ikeda, *Breast Imaging: THE REQUISITES*, p 285.

Comment

This patient presented with a palpable mass while she was nursing. A limited mammogram was performed, which demonstrated a very dense breast. The main reason for performing a mammogram in this situation is to check for microcalcifications. Ideally, the workup of a young woman who presents with a palpable lump during pregnancy or lactation should begin with ultrasound. If the ultrasound exam is normal, a single MLO view can be performed to exclude the presence of microcalcifications.

This example demonstrates the marked change in breast parenchyma during and after lactation. The glandular tissue during lactation is extremely dense, and masses may be obscured, reducing the sensitivity of the exam.

Notes

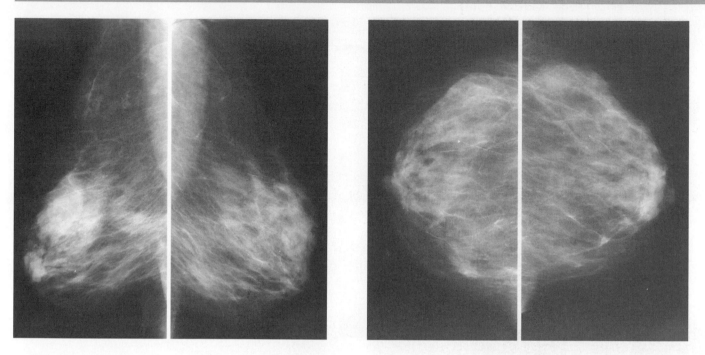

1. This baseline mammogram is not optimally positioned. Critique the MLO views in terms of the quality of the positioning.

2. Critique the cranial caudad views in terms of positioning.

3. What is the nipple-to-pectoralis line?

4. What BI-RADS category and recommendation should be given?

CASE 9

Poor Positioning, Missed Cancer

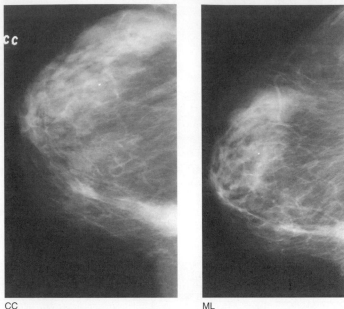

CC   ML

1. In the MLO views, the breasts are drooping and there is poor visualization of the pectoralis muscle and posterior breast.

2. The cranial caudad views are short, particularly the left CC view.

3. The nipple-to-pectoralis line (NPL) is a measurement on the MLO view from the nipple straight back to the edge of the muscle, perpendicular to the axis of the pectoralis. The NPL length measured on the MLO view is then compared to the nipple to film edge on the cranial caudad view. The distance on the CC view from nipple back to the film edge (or the depth of breast tissue imaged on the CC view) should be no less than 1 cm of the NPL measured on the MLO view. In this case, the comparison of the NPL on the MLO view to the CC view shows that the CC views are quite short.

4. This case should be given a BI-RADS category 0, incomplete, and the patient should be a "technical callback." The patient should be recalled and adequate imaging performed at no charge.

References

Eklund GW, Cardenosa G: The art of mammographic positioning, *Radiol Clin North Am* 30(1):21–53, 1992.

Majid AS, Shaw de Paredes E, Doherty RD, Sharma NR, Salvador X: Missed breast carcinoma: Pitfalls and pearls, *RadioGraphics* 23:881–895, 2003.

Cross-Reference

Ikeda, *Breast Imaging: THE REQUISITES*, p 6.

Comment

Adequate positioning requires diligence on the part of the radiology technologist and cooperation by the patient. In this case, the breasts are sagging on the MLO views, and there is poor visualization of the posterior breast tissue. In addition, the pectoralis muscles are not seen extending to at least the nipple level on the MLO views because the breasts are drooping. The pectoralis muscles should also ideally bulge convexly toward the nipple demonstrating that the breasts have been pulled up and out for the MLO views. It is obvious that a large amount of breast tissue is not well imaged on the MLO views. In addition, the cranial caudad views are quite short compared to the nipple-to-pectoral distance on the MLO views. Significantly more breast tissue is seen on the technically limited medial lateral oblique views than is seen on the cranial caudad views; the difference between the nipple-to-pectoralis distance on the MLO views and the nipple to the posterior edge of the film on the cranial caudad views is more than 3 cm.

The patient was recalled and improved imaging was performed. With the improved imaging, a 2-cm cancer was evident in the medial left breast. If the radiologist had accepted the technically suboptimal initial study, this large tumor would have been missed. Although "perfect" images cannot be obtained on all patients, it is very important to maintain a standard of imaging that is reproducible and diagnostic.

Notes

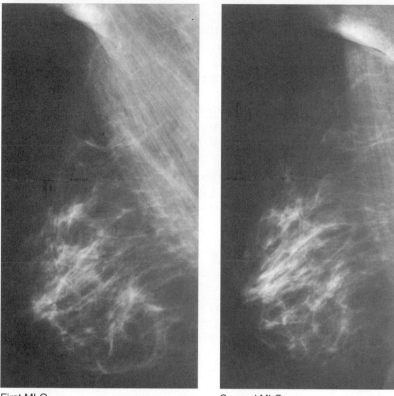

First MLO   Second MLO

1. The MLO view on the left has poorly seen calcifications in the inferior breast. The repeat image is on the right. Describe the findings.

2. Why are the calcifications not seen well on the first image?

3. Where is motion unsharpness most likely to occur, and on which images?

4. What are the causes of motion unsharpness?

Motion on MLO—Calcifications

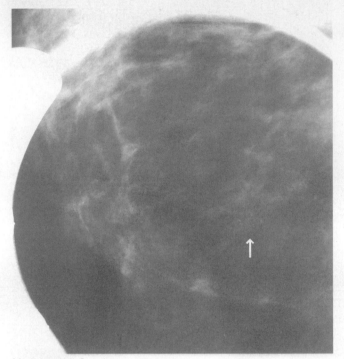

Motion on MLO, calcs

1. There is a cluster of heterogeneous calcifications seen in a linear distribution.

2. There is motion unsharpness.

3. Motion occurs most often in the inferior breast on MLO views.

4. Prolonged exposures, poor compression, and patient motion.

References

Bassett LW: Clinical image evaluation, *Radiol Clin North Am* 33(6):1027–1039, 1995.

Eklund GW, Cardenosa G: The art of mammographic positioning, *Radiol Clin North Am* 30(1):21–53, 1992.

Majid AS, Shaw de Paredes E, Doherty RD, Sharma NR, Salvador X: Missed breast carcinoma: Pitfalls and pearls, *RadioGraphics* 23:881–895, 2003.

Cross-Reference

Ikeda, *Breast Imaging: THE REQUISITES*, p 6.

Comment

This case demonstrates motion unsharpness in the inferior breast on the MLO view. The repeat image reveals heterogeneous calcifications in the inferior breast that on biopsy were due to DCIS. The motion unsharpness is due to poor positioning and undercompression. This type of motion unsharpness frequently occurs in the inferior aspect of the breast on the MLO view. In this case, inadequate compression is evident by the overlapping and sagging breast tissues in the inferior breast. The inframmary fold is not open, and the breast is not pulled "up and out." Proper compression reduces breast thickness and reduces the dose needed for a proper exposure. Therefore, contrast is improved by decreasing scatter radiation. Adequate compression also immobilizes the breast and decreases the likelihood of motion unsharpness, as in this example. If the initial MLO had not been repeated, the calcifications of DCIS may have been missed by the radiologist.

Notes

1. This patient presents for a routine mammogram. The asymmetric density in the left breast is stable over many years. The BB marker on the left CC view indicates a mole. The marker is not seen on MLO view. What does this tell you?

2. Why are BB markers placed on moles?

3. Is it possible that a breast cancer could be seen only on the CC view and not on the MLO view?

4. Is positioning the responsibility of the radiologist or the technologist?

Positioning—Mole

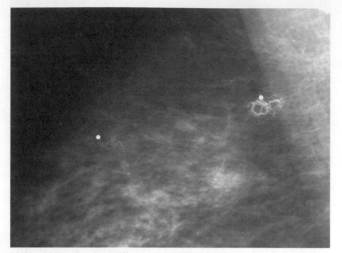

Mole with marker in a different patient

1. The standard MLO view may miss structures in the medial aspect of the breast. The mole is in the medial aspect of the left breast.

2. Moles are marked so they are not confused with possible breast mass.

3. Yes, a cancer may be seen only on the CC view, not included in the MLO view because of extreme medial location.

4. The radiologist bears the ultimate responsibility for image quality. If the technologist is not properly positioning the patient, more training is needed.

Reference

Eklund GW, Cardenosa G: The art of mammographic positioning, *Radiol Clin North Am* 30(1):21–53, 1992.

Cross-Reference

Ikeda, *Breast Imaging: THE REQUISITES*, p 26.

Comment

The MLO view was designated as the standard view of the breast instead of a straight sagittal, or ML view, because it better visualizes the upper outer quadrant of the breast. Most of a woman's glandular breast tissue, and thus most breast cancer, is located in the upper outer quadrant. However, cancer may be located in any part of the breast, and masses seen in the far medial aspect are not unusual.

The MLO view may miss some of the medial aspect of the breast. In order to compensate for this, the CC view should be positioned to include as much medial tissue as possible without rotating the nipple from the midline. Far lateral tissue may not be completely included on the CC view, and additional "exaggerated CC" views may be needed to completely visualize the lateral breast tissue.

Notes

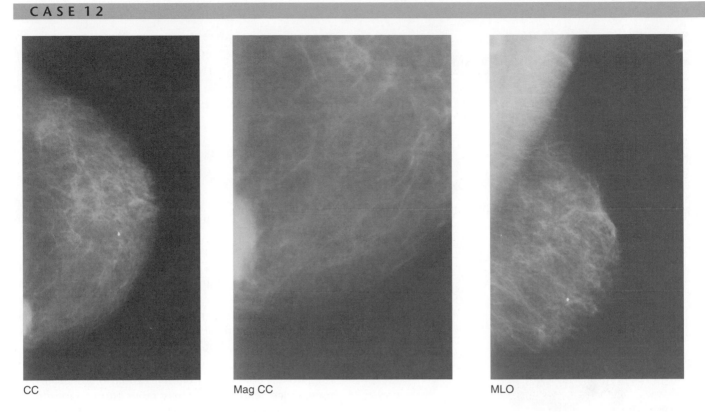

CC   Mag CC   MLO

1. There is a focal asymmetry along the posterior medial edge of the cranial caudal view. What is this structure?

2. Is further workup needed?

3. Is this most often unilateral or bilateral?

4. How often is this variant found in cadaveric studies?

Sternalis

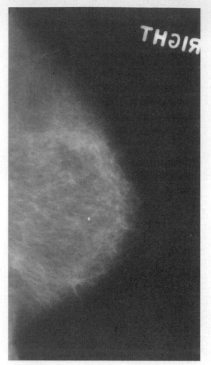

ML view

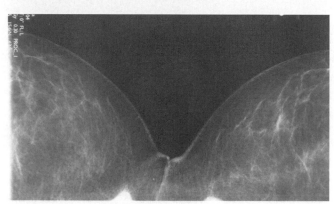

Cleavage view

1. The sternalis muscle.

2. No. This is a normal variant.

3. This is more often seen as a unilateral structure than a bilateral one. However, with improved positioning, the sternalis muscle may be seen more often.

4. Approximately 8% of the time.

Reference
Bradley FM, Hoover HC Jr, Hulka CA, Whitman GJ, McCarthy KA, Hall DA, Moore R, Kopans DB: The sternalis muscle: An unusual normal finding seen on mammography. *Am J Roentgenol* 166(1):33–36, 1996.

Cross-Reference
Ikeda, *Breast Imaging: THE REQUISITES*, p 26.

Comment
The sternalis muscle is an uncommon variant of the chest wall musculature that may be seen mammographically and misinterpreted as a mass or tumor. This thin slip of muscle runs longitudinally along the medial border of the sternum. With deep positioning on a cranial caudad view, it may be seen in the very medial aspect of the breast as a density with an ill-defined margin. The sternalis, when present, lies just anterior to the medial margin of the pectoralis muscle. It may be unilateral or bilateral, but it is not able to be reproduced on the MLO or ML view of the breast because of its thin longitudinal course in a cranial caudal orientation. The appearance of the muscle may range from an irregularly rounded density to a flame-shaped density. Usually, the focal asymmetry is surrounded by fat, causing it to stand out on the CC views. Rarely, CT or MRI may be necessary to confirm that this is indeed normal musculature, but ultrasound may also be helpful to exclude a medial mass. With improved mammographic positioning, this variant may be seen more frequently. Occasionally, when it is seen unilaterally, the patient may be positioned for a cleavage view (or "valley view") and symmetric bilateral sternalis muscles may be seen as shown above. Knowledge of the variety of appearance of this normal variant is important so that unnecessary biopsies and additional workups are avoided.

Notes

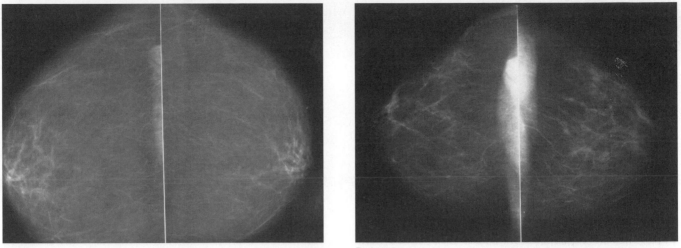

Patient 1   Patient 2

1. In the first image, there is a rounded mass seen adjacent to the chest wall in the lateral aspect of the left breast on CC. No suspicious lesion was seen on the MLO. Is this a mass or the pectoralis?

2. Is it desirable to position the breast in such a way that the pectoralis is included on the CC view?

3. In the second image, on a different patient, a double density is seen within the posterior aspect of the pectoralis only on the CC view. Is there a breast mass superimposed on the muscle?

4. What can you do in case you are not sure whether the density is a portion of the muscle?

Pectoralis Muscle on CC View of Mammogram

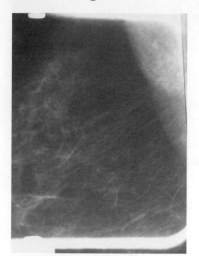

Spot compression

1. This is a portion of the pectoralis muscle.

2. It is important to position the breast as deeply as possible. If the pectoralis is seen, you can be confident that all the posterior breast tissue is included.

3. This is probably a portion of the pectoralis muscle rather than a breast mass because no mass is seen on the MLO.

4. Perform a spot compression view, with the position exaggerated to include more lateral tissue. This is shown in the image on this page, and it is easier to see that the density in question is contiguous with the muscle and does not represent a breast mass.

Reference
Eklund GW, Cardenosa G: The art of mammographic positioning, *Radiol Clin North Am* 30:21–53, 1992.

Cross-Reference
Ikeda, *Breast Imaging: THE REQUISITES*, p 26.

Comment
The pectoralis muscle lies posterior to the breast, forming the only part of the chest wall that is visualized on the mammogram. Positioning the breast in such a way so as to include as much of the breast tissue as possible is one of the most important roles of the technologist. Recognizing that as much of the breast as possible has been included on the film is one of the most important jobs of the radiologist interpreting mammograms.

A valuable tool in recognizing the adequacy of positioning is the pectoralis muscle. It should be seen on the MLO view to the level of the nipple, and it should have a convex anterior margin. On the CC view, some of the pectoralis muscle can be seen along the posterior aspect of the breast in approximately 25% of patients. When it is seen, you may be confident that the breast tissue is completely seen because the pectoralis is the most posterior structure that can be seen on the mammogram.

The pectoralis muscle may have a convex anterior margin to such an extent that it appears like a mass. Care must be taken to recognize the pectoralis muscle and yet not miss a possible mass at the edge of the film. If not sure, spot compression view may help to more completely evaluate the pectoralis muscle.

Notes

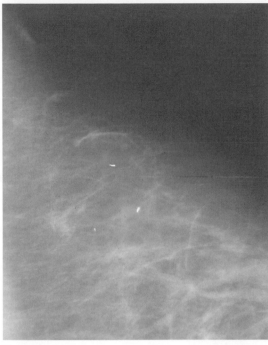

Mag view

1. A white spot is seen on the MLO view in the superior breast. There is surrounding focal unsharpness. What is this artifact due to?

2. What is the next step to resolve this problem?

3. How do you know what to clean?

4. How often should these be cleaned?

Artifacts—Film Screen Contact

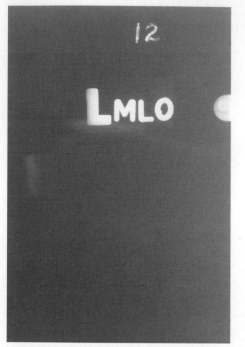

Mag of cassette markers

1. The artifact is due to a particle of dust or debris located between the film and the screen in the cassette.

2. The next step is to clean off the debris from the specific screen.

3. You must find the number of the screen on the film. It is clearly marked in the periphery of the image (#12) above the side (L) and view (MLO) in this case.

4. The screen must be cleaned weekly at a minimum.

References

Bassett LW, Hirbawi IA, DeBruhl N, Hayes MK: Mammographic positioning: Evaluation from the view box, *Radiology* 188:803–806, 1993.

Hogge JP, Palmer CH, Muller CC, Little ST, Smith DC, Fatouros PP, Shaw de Paredes E: Quality assurance in mammography: Artifact analysis, *RadioGraphics* 19:503–522, 1999.

Cross-Reference

Ikeda, *Breast Imaging: THE REQUISITES*, p 14.

Comment

The artifact, which appears as a high-density speck, is seen on the MLO image and is due to a piece of dust or debris that is positioned between the film and the screen in the cassette. The focal unsharpness surrounding the radiopaque artifact is due to the fact the film is slightly lifted off the screen by the piece of debris. To remove the artifact from the system, the cassette must be cleaned. In this case, four images were taken with four different cassettes. An identifying number unique to each cassette is found at the corner of the film so that locating the specific cassette with the artifact (#12, in this case) is easy. The technologist quickly knows which cassette to clean. Cleaning of the cassettes is a part of the maintenance quality control program that must be performed in a mammography department. The cassettes and screens are required to be cleaned weekly at a minimum.

Notes

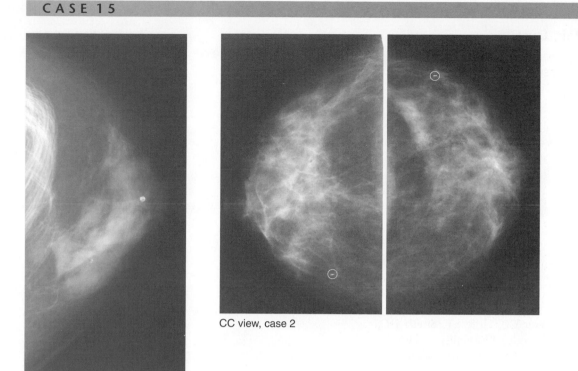

CC view, case 2

CC view, case 1

1. An artifact is seen against the chest wall in the cranial caudal view of case 1. What is this artifact?

2. What is necessary to complete this study?

3. Case 2 shows a linear high-density speck (*circle*) that was seen on all four images of the study. Where is this artifact most likely located?

4. What is the next step?

More Artifacts—Hair, Dust

1. The artifact in case 1 is a curl of hair. The swirling appearance seen against the chest wall is due to the patient's shoulder-length hair projecting over the breast during the exposure.

2. A repeat cranial caudad view should be performed to ensure that the breast tissue is entirely visible and that no finding is obscured in the posterior breast.

3. The fact that the speck appears in the same location on all images of case 2 suggests that it is on the bucky.

4. The bucky should be carefully evaluated and cleaned.

Reference

Hogge JP, Palmer CH, Muller CC, Little ST, Smith DC, Fatouros PP, Shaw de Paredes S: Quality assurance in mammography: Artifact analysis, *RadioGraphics* 19:503–522, 1999.

Cross-Reference

Ikeda, *Breast Imaging: THE REQUISITES*, pp 6, 72.

Comment

Identification of artifacts is important in high-quality imaging. Artifacts should not be confused for suspicious findings, nor should they be overlooked. In the case of the curl of hair, faint calcifications could be obscured in the posterior breast. The hair is due to the patient turning her head and her shoulder-length hair flipping over her shoulder into the beam during the exposure. This artifact is frequently seen laterally on the cranial caudal projection as the patient turns her head away from the breast during the positioning. This artifact is rarely seen on MLO views.

The small linear radial opacity is obviously an artifact. It appears in the same location relative to the film flash in all four projections. Since a different cassette is used for each of the four images, the artifact must be separate from the film, screen, and cassette. This finding is most likely a piece of lint or debris on the bucky or compression plate. Because of the sharpness, it is most likely closest to the cassette and on the bucky. If it were unsharp, the artifact would more likely be the superior or medial plastic compression plate on the cranial caudal and MLO views, respectively. Inspection of the bucky and cleaning are needed. Both the compression plates and the surface of the bucky should be cleaned after each use.

Notes

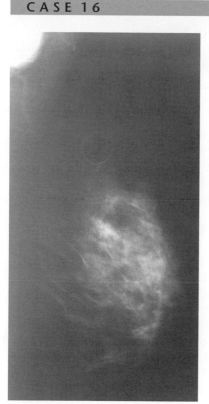

First MLO

1. On this baseline screening, a finding was seen on the right MLO view. Describe the finding in the right axilla.

2. What BI-RADS category should be given for this screening study?

3. What is the next image to be performed?

4. What is the most likely diagnosis following the additional imaging?

Artifacts—Chin

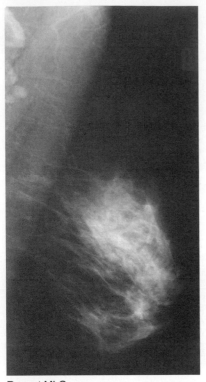

Repeat MLO

1. A large radiopaque focal asymmetry or mass is seen high in the axilla.

2. On this screening study, a BI-RADS "category 0: incomplete, additional imaging needed" is appropriate.

3. The next step would be to repeat the MLO view. A deeper projection should be obtained with better positioning to show more of the pectoralis muscle extending to the nipple level.

4. On repeat imaging, there is no mass. The "pseudo-mass" was due to the chin projecting over the high axilla in the oblique projection.

References

Bassett LW, Hirbawi IA, DeBruhl N, Hayes MK: Mammographic positioning: Evaluation from the view box, *Radiology* 188:803–806, 1993.

Eklund GW, Cardenosa G: The art of mammographic positioning, *Radiol Clin North Am* 30(1):21–53, 1992.

Cross-Reference

Ikeda, *Breast Imaging: THE REQUISITES,* p 72.

Comment

On first glance, there appears to be a large mass high in the axilla. This could possibly be a very large lymph node. However, the patient is asymptomatic. On inspection, the margin is slightly irregular and unsharp, suggesting that the focal asymmetry is actually artifactual. The MLO view is obtained in a 45° obliquity, and if the patient is not positioned carefully, the chin may project over the axilla and axillary tail, particularly in a woman with a kyphosis. The next step would be to repeat the MLO view with the chin in a position in which it will not project over the breast during the exposure. The repeat image shows complete resolution of the mass and deeper imaging of the axilla. This type of case is called a technical callback, and the patient should not be charged for the additional imaging since the images should have been checked by the technologist for quality prior to the departure of the patient from the screening facility. A diligent technologist should catch this finding and know that it is purely artifactual due to the chin projecting into the beam of exposure. The technologist should have repeated the additional MLO prior to the patient departing the facility.

Notes

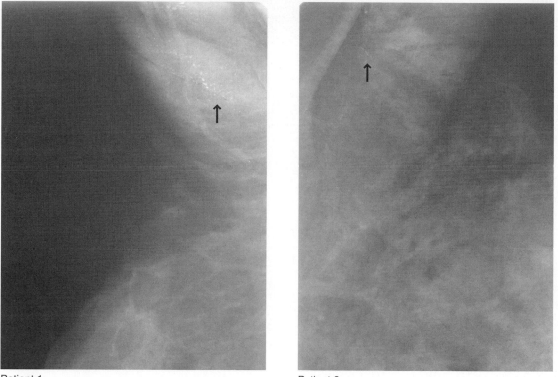

Patient 1   Patient 2

1. Two magnification MLO views of the axillae of two different patients are shown. Describe the findings.

2. What is the next recommendation?

3. What ingredients in deodorant create this appearance?

4. What other compounds may cause this appearance?

Artifacts—Deodorant

1. The small radiopaque particles in the axilla may represent deodorant.

2. The patient should be instructed to carefully cleanse the axilla, and repeat views should be obtained. If the small radiopacities do not entirely resolve, careful imaging for triangulation is necessary. On the left, the particles are deodorant. On the right, the calcifications are due to DCIS.

3. Antiperspirants and deodorants may contain metallic compounds including aluminum.

4. Other powders, cremes, ointments, or tatoos may contain radiopaque material that may mimic suspicious calcifications.

References

Bassett LW, Jackson VP, Jahan R, Fu YS, Gold RH: *Diagnosis of Diseases of the Breast*, Philadelphia, 1997, Saunders, pp 363–364.

Hogge JP, Palmer CH, Muller CC, Little ST, Smith DC, Fatouros PP, Shaw de Paredes E: Quality assurance in mammography: Artifact analysis, *RadioGraphics* 19:503–522, 1999.

Cross-Reference

Ikeda, *Breast Imaging*: THE REQUISITES, p 70.

Comment

A number of materials that are applied to the skin may be radiopaque. Most commonly seen is underarm deodorant or antiperspirant that contains a metallic compound that includes aluminum. Many deodorants do not contain metallic material and are not visible mammographically. Many mammographic facilities suggest that patients not wear deodorant on the day of their studies, or if they do use deodorant, cleansing towels are provided for the patient. It is frequently quite easy to differentiate the metallic compound due to antiperspirant because it follows the skin lines or wrinkles of the axilla. However, occasionally, cleansing is needed to exclude suspicious calcifications in the axilla. The image on the right shows such a case. Despite cleansing, these linear and pleomorphic calcifications persisted. On breast biopsy, these calcifications were due to ductal carcinoma *in situ* in breast tissue high in the axilla.

Other materials that are applied to the skin may appear very radiopaque. Skin powders, cremes, or ointments may have compounds that may mimic suspicious microcalcifications mammographically. Tangential imaging should show that the radiopaque material is within the skin, and then cleansing would be recommended.

Notes

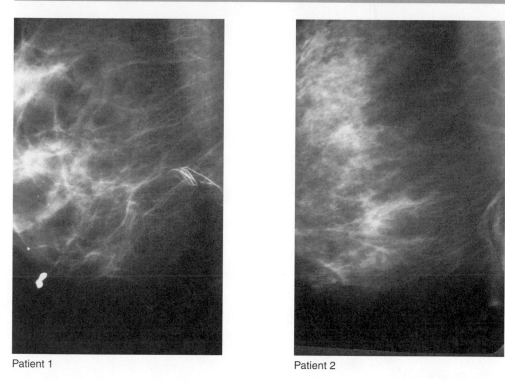

Patient 1   Patient 2

1. What is the structure in the lower left breast near the chest wall in these two different patients?

2. Is this structure in the breast or an artifact?

3. Is this artifact related to processing issues or to the patient?

4. How can this be avoided?

Artifact on Mammogram—Gown

1. The structure is linear positive density that does not correspond to the anatomic arrangement of breast tissue.

2. The structure is not related to the breast, so it must be an artifact.

3. Processing problems are specks, lines, static, and fingerprints. This is on the patient.

4. The technologist's responsibility is to check for hair, clothing, and anything on the skin between the breast and the mammographic unit prior to compressing the breast.

Reference

Hogge JP, Palmer CH, Muller CC, Little ST, Smith DC, Fatouros PP, Shaw de Paredes, E: Quality assurance in mammography: Artifact analysis, *RadioGraphics* 19:503–522, 1999.

Cross-Reference

Ikeda, *Breast Imaging: THE REQUISITES*, p 6.

Comment

Artifacts can be thought of as abnormalities in density on the mammogram that do not belong to the breast. They may be caused by any event during the mammogram process. Often, there are structures between the breast and the back support, or film holder, caught in that position during compression and not noticed by the technologist. Jewelry is easy to recognize because it causes a metal density artifact. Hair has a distinctive appearance, consisting of faint linear densities that should not be confused with calcification.

In this example, the artifact is a string from the cloth gown she is wearing. The technologist will see the string if it is between the breast and the clear plastic compression paddle, so this must be on the far side of the breast, between the breast and the opaque film holder. Ideally, the technologist, when checking the images after they are processed and prior to sending the patient home, will check for artifacts and repeat views when artifacts are present.

Notes

1. What do you notice on the medial aspect of the CC views of both breasts?

2. Is biopsy indicated?

3. Is there anything else in the differential diagnosis?

4. The pattern of the tiny densities is helpful in the diagnosis. Describe the pattern.

Artifact on Skin

1. There are very tiny densities on the film.

2. This is not microcalcification, although the x-ray density is similar to calcium. Biopsy is not indicated.

3. In the differential diagnosis is talc or lotion on the skin, which becomes trapped in skin irregularities.

4. The pattern is round groups of tiny densities on the medial aspect of the breast.

References

Barton JW III, Kornguth PJ: Mammographic deodorant and powder artifact: Is there confusion with malignant microcalcifications? *Breast Dis* 3:121–126, 1990.

Pamilo M, Soiva M, Suramo I: New artifacts simulating malignant microcalcifications in mammography, *Breast Dis* 1:321–327, 1989.

Cross-Reference

Ikeda, *Breast Imaging: THE REQUISITES*, p 70.

Comment

Patients often apply lotions and deodorants on the skin. Patients should be asked to refrain from using deodorant, lotions, and powders prior to their mammogram. Some products, particularly thick ointments, may remain on the skin after washing. This was the case with this patient, who used a product on her skin similar to diaper rash ointment because of irritation of the skin under the breasts. Her skin had multiple small round moles, and the skin ointment was trapped in the irregular surface of the moles, causing the artifact on the film.

You may ask the patient to vigorously wash the skin when you see this artifact, or you may visually inspect the skin for the small skin moles that trap the lotion. This artifact is similar in appearance to deodorant on the skin of the axillae; both can be confused with microcalcification.

Notes

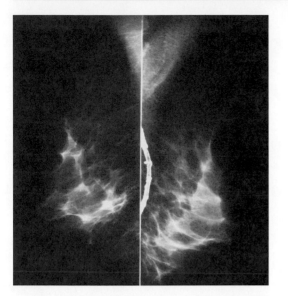

1. The abnormality is the tubular-shaped calcified structure in the right breast. What could cause this?
2. If this is artifact, is it in the patient or on the patient?
3. The technologist reports that there is nothing on the patient's skin. Now what?
4. Would old films be useful?

Artifact—VP Shunt

1. This is unlikely to be calcification caused by vascular or ductal structures because it is so regular and is very thick and densely calcified. It looks man-made.

2. The patient must be checked to determine if there is an artifact on the skin.

3. The calcified structure must be in the patient's body. A careful history may give the diagnosis.

4. Old films are always useful. In this case, the calcified structure was seen on prior films for many years. The patient has a ventriculoperitoneal shunt.

Reference

Hogge JP, Palmer CH, Muller CC, Little ST, Smith DC, Fatouros PP, Shaw de Paredes, E: Quality assurance in mammography: Artifact analysis, *RadioGraphics* 19:503–522, 1999.

Cross-Reference

Ikeda, *Breast Imaging: THE REQUISITES*, p 6.

Comment

Artifacts are abnormalities in mammographic density that are not native to the breast. Artifacts can occur in any component of the imaging process. Artifacts related to the patient can be due to motion or due to superimposed objects, such as deodorant, lotion, hair, jewelry, and implanted medical devices. In this case, the patient has a vetriculoperitoneal shunt for hydrocephalus, and the tubing is seen on the mammogram.

In this patient, the shunt tubing is calcified, but this shunt may be seen without calcification.

Notes

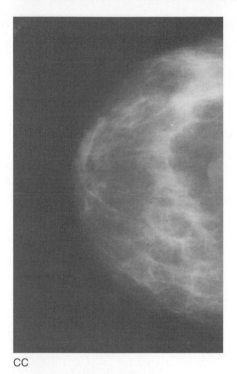

CC

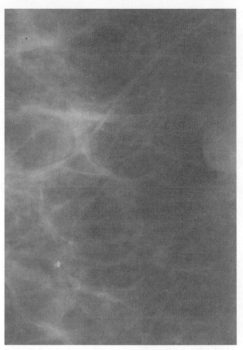

Mag CC

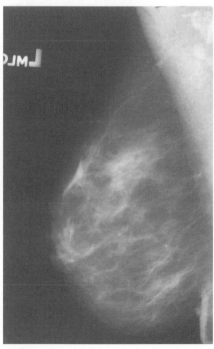

MLO

1. This patient has a partially well-circumscribed mass seen centrally on the CC view and inferiorly, near the inframammary fold on the MLO view. What is the differential diagnosis?

2. What is the next diagnostic step?

3. In what other locations may a similar finding be seen?

4. How common is this finding?

Accessory Nipple

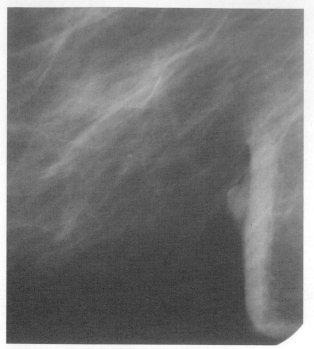

Mag MLO of inferior breast

1. The location and the sharp, air-marginated anterior squared-off shape of this mass are almost pathognomonic for an accessory nipple. A sebaceous cyst could also be in the differential diagnosis.

2. Look at the patient questionnaire or find out if the technologist noticed a skin lesion. If uncertain, the patient should be examined and, if necessary, a metallic BB could be placed on the skin lesion.

3. Where the "milk line" occurs.

4. Up to 6% of women will have some form of accessory breast tissue.

Reference

Samardar P, Shaw de Paredes E, Grimes MM, Wilson JD: Focal asymmetric densities seen at mammography: US and pathologic correlation, *RadioGraphics* 22: 19–33, 2002.

Cross-Reference

Ikeda, *Breast Imaging: THE REQUISTES*, p 37.

Comment

Incomplete regression or remnants of the primitive milk line may lead to accessory mounds or supernumerary nipples in approximately 2–6% of adult women, and occasionally a mass or focal asymmetry will be seen mammographically. Frequently, women are not actually aware of the presence of the supernumerary nipple because the skin lesion looks more like a freckle or mole rather than a fully developed plateau-type nipple. The supernumerary nipples may appear anywhere along the milk line that extends from the axilla to groin. Occasionally, breast tissue will become evident under the supernumerary nipple, particularly when a woman becomes pregnant.

Notes

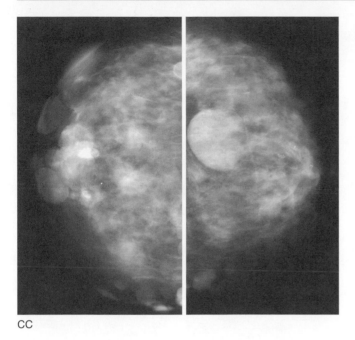

CC

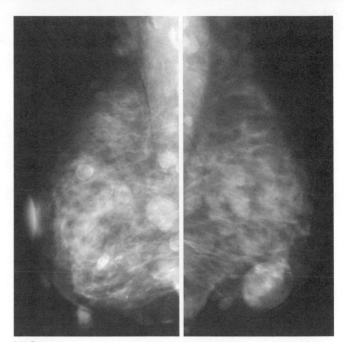

MLO

1. Describe the bilateral breast findings.

2. What is the most likely cause of these masses?

3. Is there an increased incidence of malignancies in these patients?

4. What is the BI-RADS category?

Neurofibromatosis

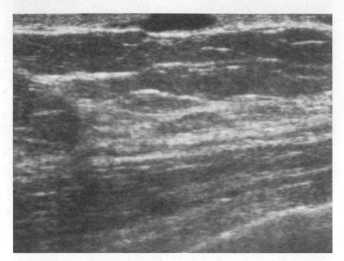

1. Bilateral well-circumscribed masses, which on close inspection are skin lesions.

2. Neurofibromatosis.

3. Although the literature varies, there does appear to be an increased incidence of malignancies in these patients.

4. BI-RADS category 2: benign.

References

el-Zawahry MD, Farid M, Abd el-Latif A, Horeia H, el-Gindy M, Twakal G: Breast lesions in generalized neurofibromatosis: Breast cancer and cystosarcoma phylloides, *Neurofibromatosis* 2(2):121–124, 1989.

Millman SL, Mercado CL: An unusual presentation of neurofibromatosis of the breast, *Breast J* 10(1):45, 2004.

Cross-Reference

Ikeda, *Breast Imaging: THE REQUISITES*, p 315.

Comment

This patient has neurofibromatosis or von Recklinghausen's disease. There are two distinct forms of neurofibromatosis: type 1 (NF1) and type 2 (NF2). NF1 is more common and is characterized by multiple skin neurofibromas, café-au-lait spots, bone defects, visual disorders, and spinal cord neurofibromas. The disorder may be either inherited in an autosomal dominant manner or occur sporadically. NF is a consequence of abnormal differentiation and migration of neural cells during the early stages of embryogenesis.

In this case, the mammogram reveals multiple round masses that are at least partially outlined by air causing sharp margins. The definition of the borders of these margins is lost where the peduculated masses attach to the skin. Frequently, the breasts are difficult to evaluate on mammography due to the numerous masses, and through imaging is necessary because these patients often have a very difficult clinical exam. If there is concern over any mass not being on the skin, metallic markers may be placed and ultrasound may be necessary. Ultrasound images, if performed, may show intracutaneous lesions, as in this case. Care must be taken to adjust the focal zones and depth of the ultrasound to image the near field as well as the deeper tissue to exclude concomitant breast lesions.

Benign and malignant neoplasms occur in excess in patients with NF1, but estimates vary greatly. The incidence of sarcomatous change of neurofibromas varies from 2–16%.

Notes

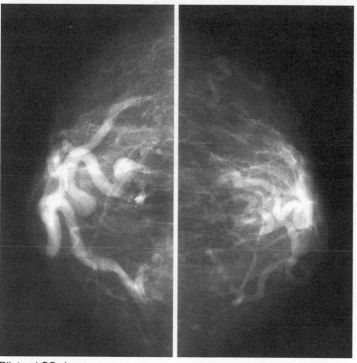

Bilateral CC views

1. What is the appropriate BI-RADS term to describe the mammographic findings?

2. What is the differential diagnosis?

3. What BI-RADS category is given?

4. Are there any management recommendations?

SVC Syndrome

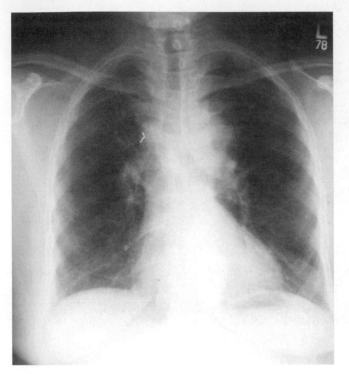

Other causes of complete or partial obstruction of the superior vena cava include mediastinal tumors such as lymphoma, adenocarcinoma of the lung, and other large mediastinal masses. Less common causes include chronic fibrotic mediastinitis, either idiopathic or due to granulomateous diseases or drugs. Symptoms other than dilated chest wall vasculature may include swelling of the face and neck, visual disturbances, and headaches. If the venous dilatation from SVC obstruction is unilateral, it is more often seen in the right breast. Rarely, superficially dilated venous structures may be seen with no known underlying cause. In this case the chest x-ray shows fullness in the mediastinal due to extensive collateral venous structures. Physical exam and clinical correlation are recommended to determine if an underlying etiology may be treatable.

Notes

1. This a case of bilaterally (slightly asymmetric) dilated veins.

2. There are no suspicious breast findings and presumably the dilated venous structures are due to obstructed vessels with venous collateral formation.

3. This should be a BI-RADS category 2: benign.

4. A call to the referring physician to make sure he or she is aware of the venous obstruction and understands any clinical findings.

Reference

Bassett LW, Jackson VP, Jahan R, Fu YS, Gold RH: *Diagnosis of Diseases of the Breast*, Philadelphia, 1997, Saunders.

Cross-Reference

Ikeda, *Breast Imaging: THE REQUISITES*, p 299.

Comment

Dilated vascular structures may be seen mammographically in situations in which collateral blood flow develops. In this patient, the development of collateral flow was due to superior vena caval obstruction due to multiple bilateral indwelling catheters causing thrombophlebitis. The obstruction and collateral formation presumably are compensated since there is no evidence of breast or chest wall edema in this patient.

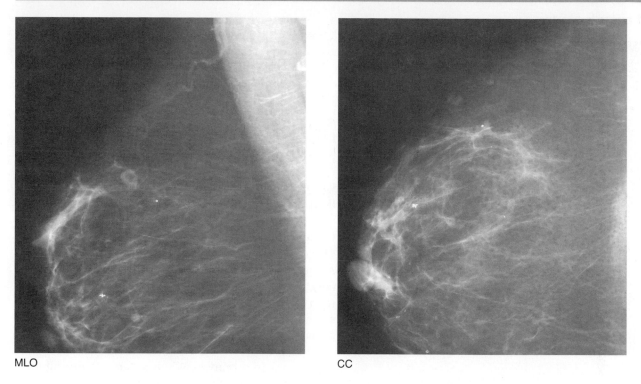

MLO   CC

1. On a baseline screening mammogram, a small mass is seen in the upper left breast. Describe the findings.

2. What BI-RADS category is given?

3. Where are these types of masses most commonly located?

4. Describe the ultrasound findings.

Normal Lymph Nodes

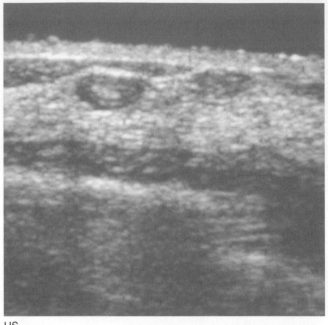

US

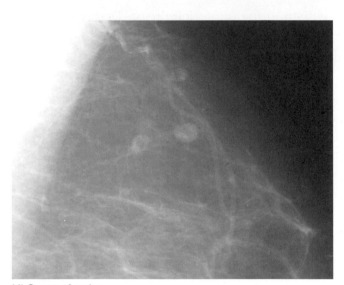

MLO mag of nodes

1. A small well-defined mass with a central fatty hilum is seen in the upper outer quadrant. This is a benign-appearing intramammary lymph node. The mass is seen along the course of a blood vessel.

2. BI-RADS category 1 or 2.

3. Lymph nodes are most commonly seen in the axilla extending into the axillary tail of the lateral breast. Less commonly, they may be seen in the superior central breast and rarely inferiorly in the breast.

4. On ultrasound, a normal intramammary lymph node will have a very well-defined margin with a hyperechoic central fatty hilum. Frequently, a nearby blood vessel is seen with flow entering the fatty hilum.

Reference

Leibman AJ, Wong R: Findings on mammography in the axilla, *Am J Roentgenol* 169(5):1385–1390, 1997.

Cross-Reference

Ikeda, *Breast Imaging: THE REQUISITES*, p 26.

Comment

This is a very common finding on a mammogram. Additional imaging evaluation to demonstrate a central fatty hilum makes one feel comfortable that this is a normal intramammary lymph node. Lymph nodes are most commonly seen in the axilla extending into the axillary tail. When seen in the breast, they are frequently located along a blood vessel, similar to an apple on a tree branch. When a central fatty hilum is seen and there are no irregularities of the margin mammographically or changes in the size, shape, or density of the lymph node over time, a BI-RADS category 2 is appropriate. Not every lymph node must be remarked on in a report, and if they are symmetric and require no further evaluation, a BI-RADS category 1 may be sufficient.

On ultrasound, normal intramammary lymph nodes have a reniform appearance and a fatty echogenic hilum is present. Frequently with vascular imaging, blood flow can be seen entering into the fatty hilum. There should be a well-circumscribed margin and no excentric bulging or irregularities. Ultrasound is not necessary if the lymph node is stable mammographically and has the typical appearance with a visible fatty hilum. However, if a fatty hilum is not visible mammographically, an ultrasound may be helpful in identifying a fatty hilum.

Notes

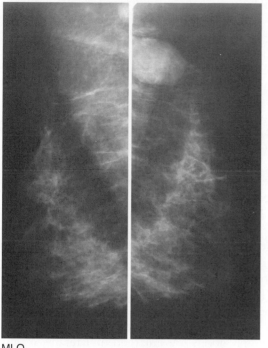

MLO

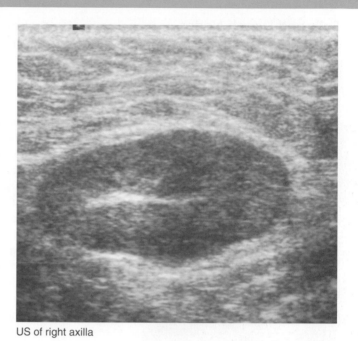

US of right axilla

1. On the baseline screening mammography study in this 45-year-old woman, a mass is seen high in the right breast on the MLO view. What additional imaging is recommended?

2. Is ultrasound necessary in this case? Describe the findings.

3. What is the differential diagnosis for bilateral enlarged lymph nodes?

4. What BI-RADS category and clinical recommendation should be given?

Bilateral Enlarged Lymph Nodes

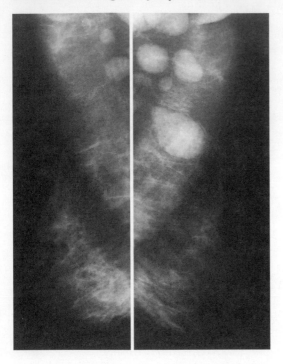

1. The appearance suggests that this is actually an enlarged low axillary lymph node. The next imaging could include deeper views of the right axilla but also of the contralateral axilla to determine if the process is bilateral.

2. Ultrasound is not necessary if you know that the mass is actually a node. Ultrasound can be helpful to guide a biopsy.

3. Bilateral enlargement of axillary nodes suggests a systemic process, such as a lymphoproliferative disorder (lymphoma or leukemia). Other etiologies include sarcoid, rheumatoid arthritis, and HIV.

4. When an extramammary etiology is determined, such as lymphoma or rheumatoid arthritis as in this case, a BI-RADS category 2, benign, is given. If there is no known etiology for the bilateral adenopathy, a category 0, incomplete, could be given in anticipation of the results of other clinical tests.

Reference

Walsh R, Kornguth PJ, Soo MS, Bentley R, DeLong DM: Axillary lymph nodes: Mammographic, pathologic, and clinical correlation, *Am J Roentgenol* 168:33–38, 1997.

Cross-Reference

Ikeda, *Breast Imaging: THE REQUISITES*, p 303.

Comment

Axillary lymph nodes or low-lying intramammary lymph nodes, often in the tail of Spence, are variable in size, number, and appearance. They generally are well-circumscribed or macrolulated masses, and frequently a fatty hilum is visuable mammographically. Careful comparison to prior mammograms to show that the size and density of the nodes are stable is necessary.

In this baseline mammogram, the multiple bilaterally enlarged lymph nodes are quite dense and no fatty hila are seen. Bilateral axillary adenopathy is most commonly due to an extramammary source such as a lymphoproliferative disorder, such as lymphoma and leukemia. In an older population, chronic lymphocytic leukemia is a common etiology. This patient has rheumatoid arthritis and the adenopathy is consistent with her disease status. Benign bilateral adenopathy may also be seen with other systemic diseases, such as lymphoid hyperplasia; granulomatous diseases, such as sarcoid and tuberculosis; other collagen vascular disorders, such as scleroderma and lupus; and HIV.

When lymph nodes are enlarged unilaterally, a unilateral breast primary must be excluded. An imaging workup, which may include MRI, is recommended and a core biopsy or FNA of the node may be needed under ultrasound guidance.

Notes

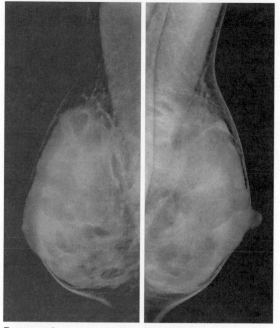

Processed   Raw image

1. Above is a screening digital mammogram of a 55-year-old woman. Does digital mammography offer improved cancer detection rates for the general population?

2. What specific subgroups of women may benefit from digital mammography rather than film screen mammography for screening according to the Digital Mammography Imaging Screening Trial (DMIST) data?

3. What is a possible reason for this difference in sensitivity?

4. Is the dose of digital mammography comparable to film screen mammography?

Digital Mammography

1. According to the results of the DMIST, there is no improvement in cancer detection rate for digital mammography over film screen mammography for the general population.

2. When subgroup analyses were performed on the DMIST data, an improvement in cancer detection was seen in three subgroups: women younger than age 50 years, women with heterogeneously dense or denser breasts, and pre- or perimenopausal women.

3. The improved contrast resolution of digital mammography is thought to contribute to improved detection of cancer in women with dense breasts (of which a higher percentage fall into the three groups mentioned previously).

4. The dose of a digital mammogram is slightly lower than that of a film screen study.

References

Pisano ED, Yaffe MJ: Digital mammography, *Radiology* 234:353–362, 2005.

Pisano ED, et al., the Digital Mammographic Imaging Screening Trial (DMIST) Investigators Group: Diagnostic performance of digital versus film mammography for breast-cancer screening, *N Engl J Med* 353:1773–1783, 2005.

Pisano ED, et al.: American College of Radiology Imaging Network Digital Mammographic Imaging Screening Trial: Objectives and methodology, *Radiology* 236:404–412, 2005.

Cross-Reference

Ikeda, *Breast Imaging: THE REQUISTES*, p 15

Comment

In 2002, the National Cancer Institute launched the $26 million Digital Mammographic Imaging Screening Trial, involving 49,528 women at 33 sites in the United States and Canada using four different digital imaging systems. In the study, women underwent both film screen and digital mammograms, and each mammogram was read independently by a different radiologist. The result of each mammogram was also acted on independently (patients were called back for additional imaging or biopsy if either or both mammograms had significant findings). In the total population of almost 50,000 women, there was no overall difference in cancer detection rates between screen film and digital mammography. However, when subgroup analyses were performed, the digital technology detected significantly more cancers than film screen in women with dense breasts, women who had not gone through menopause, and in women who were younger than age 50 years. The cancers detected by the digital technology and not by the film screen studies included a significant portion of large invasive carcinomas.

Further studies are currently under way to determine why the radiologists detected more cancers on digital mammography in these subgroups. It is well known that radiologists prefer the presentation of digital mammography due to the improved contrast resolution, and it is postulated that in women with dense breasts, this improved contrast resolution is particularly important to detect cancers that may be obscured by surrounding glandular tissue in lower contrast film screen images.

Digital mammography can be performed at a lower dose image-by-image than film screen mammography. Smaller detectors, however, may require multiple images to be "tiled" together in larger breasted women, and with increasing numbers of images on a small detector, the overall dose may be increased. In general, however, the dose for an individual digital mammographic image is less than that of a film screen image.

Notes

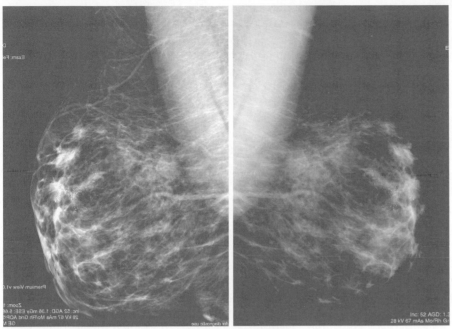

RT MLO view, processed   RT MLO view, raw

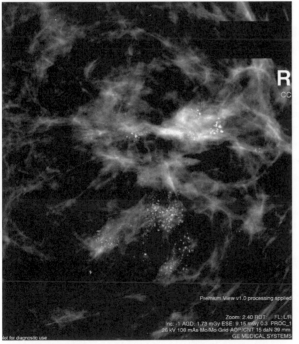

Magnified image

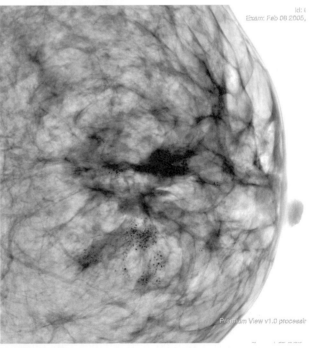

Inverted image

1. The digital mammogram of this 38-year-old woman reveals extensive calcifications in the subareolar area of the right breast. Above are right MLO projections of the right breast only. The images on the right are "raw" images. What does this mean?

2. How does the spatial resolution of digital mammography compare with film screen mammography?

3. How does the contrast resolution of digital mammography compare with film screen mammography?

4. What are some potential advantages of digital mammography?

Digital Mammography—Image Processing

1. Because the acquisition and display of digital images are separated, the image data may be manipulated prior to or during display to optimize aspects of the image. In this case, a processing algorithm has been applied that optimizes contrast and sharpness and "equalizes" the subcutaneous tissue optical densities so that the skin and immediate tissues are more visible than on the raw, unprocessed images.

2. The spatial resolution of digital systems (approximately 50–100 μm) is less than that of analog film screen systems (approximately 40 μm).

3. Contrast resolution is significantly better with digital mammography. In addition, the ability to manipulate the image at soft copy review allows the reader to optimize the contrast for the type of tissue (fatty versus denser) or lesion being evaluated.

4. Advantages of digital include electronical archiving to decrease film loss and allow electronic transmission of images to off-site areas (to operating room and referring physicians, etc.) and advanced applications including tomosynthesis, contrast mammography, and subtraction mammography.

Reference

Pisano ED, Yaffe MJ: Digital mammography, *Radiology* 234:353–362, 2005.

Cross-Reference

Ikeda, *Breast Imaging: THE REQUISITES*, p 15.

Comment

Digital mammography offers many technical advances over film screen mammography. Because the processes of image acquisition, image display, and storage are separated in digital systems, each of these important steps in image production may be optimized. With film screen mammography, the film in the cassette must serve all three functions—image capture, display, and storage. One obvious advantage to digital imaging is the reduction of the number of original films lost since additional images can be printed and images can be consistently brought up on monitors for interpretation.

The results of the DMIST trial have shown that there is an improvement in cancer detection rate with digital mammography and that this most likely is due to the improvement in contrast resolution of the digital systems. While digital systems do have a lower spatial resolution than analog systems (100 μm vs. 40 μm), the improvement in contrast resolution seems to outweigh the lower special resolution. A combination of these properties enhances the visibility of subtle contrast differences between tumors and normal background tissue. Film screen mammography is hampered by the small range of response of the film screen system and the high noise level. In addition, with digital soft copy review, the entire dynamic range of a digital image may be evaluated with window and leveling. In a single image, dense portions of the breast parenchyma as well as less dense areas of, for example, subcutaneous fat may be evaluated. Digital mammography has many other potential advantages over film screen mammography but especially when computer-aided diagnosis (CAD) algorithms are applied to the direct digital data rather than in the analog CAD systems, where the films must first be digitized. The digital CAD system saves time and money compared to the analog CAD system, and the CAD lesion markers are readily displayed on the digital soft copy display system already in use.

Other potential advantages are in the future applications of digital mammography that take advantage of the electronic capture of the digital image data. Early work in contrast mammography has begun combining vascular information with the mammographic images. Low-dose "mask" images are obtained and subtracted from each contrast medium–enhanced image. This technique may improve detection rates of subtle or otherwise occult breast lesions. Digital tomosynthesis is a technique that may also improve lesion conspicuity by reducing the mammographic image complexity due to the overlap of tissue structures. The tomosynthesis images are viewed as "stacked" images of the the breast that may be scrolled through. Telemammography is the transmission of digital electronic images by high-speed Internet, satellite, or wireless links from remote sites to more central reading areas. This transmitting of images may help provide mamographic services to remote areas and consolidate readings for improved efficiency and accuracy.

Notes

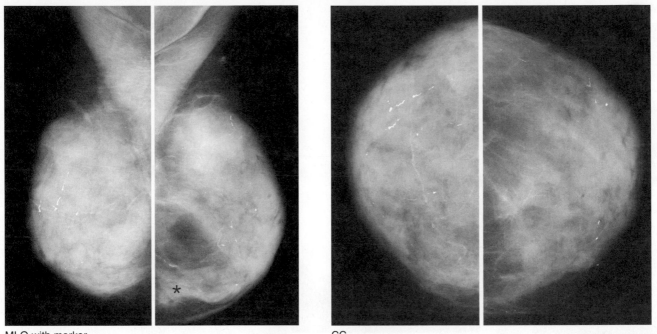

MLO with marker   CC

1. There is a subtle area of "tenting" or architectural distortion in the very inferior right breast on the MLO view (*asterisk*). Where is this most likely on the CC view?

2. What would be the next imaging step?

3. Why is it called a "spot" compression view?

4. What are the potential advantages of spot compression views?

Spot Compression View

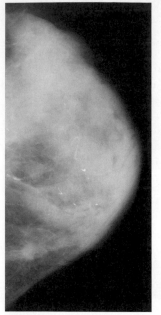

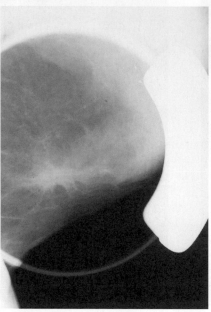

ML view

Spot mag in ML

1. To project so inferiorly in the breast on the MLO view, the potential lesion must be in the central to medial breast.

2. A spot compression view to further evaluate the area of possible distortion.

3. The "spot" refers to the small area of the breast that is compressed with a smaller paddle than used in larger area imaging. The spot increases the effective compression in a focal area.

4. Spot compression views are used to determine if a finding is "real" or just overlapping tissue. The borders of a lesion may be better defined with compression since overlapping tissue densities may be compressed and displaced.

Reference

Majid AS, Shaw de Paredes E, Doherty RD, Sharma NR, Salvador X: Missed breast carcinoma: Pitfalls and pearls, *RadioGraphics* 23:881–895, 2003.

Cross-Reference

Ikeda, *Breast Imaging: THE REQUISITES*, p 41.

Comment

The case shows a subtle area of tenting of the Cooper's ligaments in the inferior and medial right breast. The subtle change is best seen on the MLO view in the inferior breast, where the margin of breast tissue that is distorted abuts subcutaneous fat, making the subtle change more evident. When a finding is seen in only one view, the next step in imaging is to confirm that it is a real or significant finding or determine that the finding is just an illusion due to overlapping tissue structures. Often, a straight lateral view obtained in the 90° projection will provide a different image that may better demonstrate an abnormality and help triangulate a lesion if it was only seen in one of the conventional views, MLO or CC. However, spot compression views, also known as focal compression views, coned views, or spot views, are essential in working up areas of possible distortion. The spot compression view uses a small compression paddle that applies compression to a smaller area of tissue than the routine image. Therefore, the effective compression on that small region of breast is increased, which results in better tissue separation and often better visualization and the separation of normal dense areas of tissues (summation shadows) into their normal fibroglandular components. This focal compression often allows improved characterization of lesion borders and may accentuate any architectural distortion that is present. Normal glandular tissue will be displaced aside or compressed equally, whereas distortion caused by the desmoplastic growth of cancer will be accentuated, as in this case. The spot compression view shown here demonstrates a highly spiculated mass that proved to be an invasive ductal carcinoma at 5:00 in the inferior medial right breast.

Notes

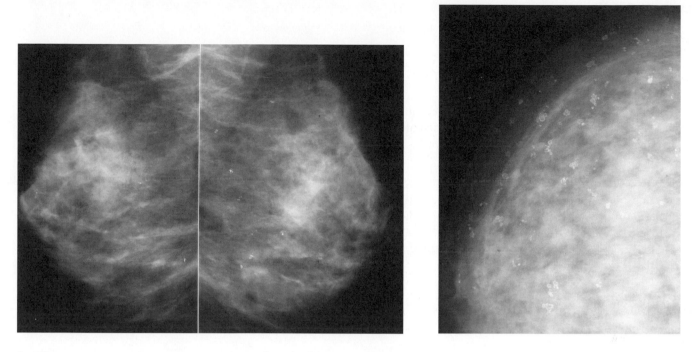

1. These are two separate patients with calcifications. What is the common feature of these two patients?

2. Are these calcifications of concern for malignancy?

3. What do the calcifications represent?

4. Do dermal calcifications always have a lucent center?

C A S E 29

Dermal Calcifications

1. Both cases have small calcifications with lucent centers.

2. These calcifications are definitely benign, BI-RADS 2.

3. These calcifications are in the skin.

4. Dermal calcifications do not have to have a lucent center. They may cluster and appear punctuate, simulating breast parenchymal calcifications.

References

American College of Radiology: *Illustrated BI-RADS*, ed 4, Reston, VA, 2004, American College of Radiology, pp 76–81.

Sickles EA: Breast calcifications: Mammographic evaluation, *Radiology* 160:289–293, 1986.

Cross-Reference

Ikeda, *Breast Imaging: THE REQUISITES*, p 73.

Comment

One of the types of benign calcifications is that of the calcification with a lucent center. This type of calcification occurs in various conditions. The small calcifications with relatively thick walls may be in the skin or can form around debris in a duct. This is the type of calcification depicted here.

When reporting calcifications, the distribution is important as well as the description of the individual shape. In skin calcifications, the distribution is usually scattered, more often seen in the peripheral aspect of the mammogram, such as the medial breast, the inframammary fold, periareolar and the axilla.

Some dermal calcifications are not lucent. Tangential views may be needed to confirm dermal location.

Notes

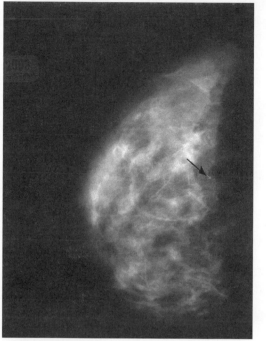

Left CC view

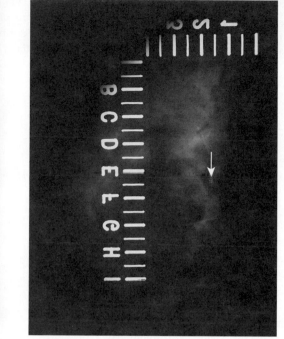

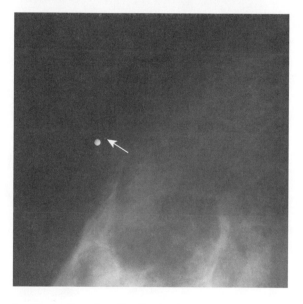

1. Describe the finding.

2. Are the calcifications benign?

3. What is the next step?

4. Should these calcifications be biopsied?

Calcifications in Skin—Localization

1. There is a grouping of calcifications in the left upper breast. The calcifications maintain the same relationship with each other in multiple views.

2. The calcifications do not fit any of the benign classifications and are considered indeterminate.

3. Because of their consistency within the group, we suspect that these represent dermal calcifications. This can be tested using the alphanumeric paddle as shown in this example.

4. Dermal calcifications need not be biopsied. They are not related to breast cancer.

References

Berkowitz JE, Gatewood OMB, Donovan GB, Gayler BW: Dermal breast calcifications: Localization with template-guided placement of skin marker, *Radiology* 163:282, 1987.

Homer MJ, D'Orsi CJ, Sitzman SB: Dermal calcifications in fixed orientation: The tattoo sign, *Radiology* 192: 161–163, 1994.

Kopans DB, Meyer JE, Homer MJ, Grabbe J: Dermal deposits mistaken for breast calcifications, *Radiology* 149:592–594, 1983.

Cross-Reference

Ikeda, *Breast Imaging: THE REQUISITES*, p 73.

Comment

Calcifications that are located in the skin are in a thin layer of dermis. They have a fixed relationship to each other, unlike calcifications seen in breast parenchyma on the mammogram. When this fixed relationship is seen on multiple views, you can easily check for the position of the calcifications in the dermal layer by a tangential view.

In order to locate the calcifications on the breast, the alphanumeric paddle used for needle localization procedures can be utilized. Place the breast in the compression device with the area of the calcifications in the window of the alphanumeric paddle. Place a BB over the location of the calcifications—in this example, between E and F and between 1 and 2. Then image the breast so that the BB is in tangent. If the calcifications are in the skin, they should be seen directly beneath the BB.

If calcifications are in the skin, the patient can be reassured that there is no increased chance of malignancy, and the calcifications do not need to be followed. She can return to routine screening. Calcifications in the skin never represent primary breast malignancy.

Skin calcifications often have a radiolucent center with thin calcific rim. When seen, these calcifications can be confidently assigned to the benign category, and tangential views are not necessary.

Notes

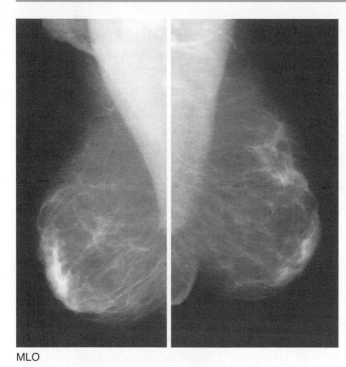

MLO

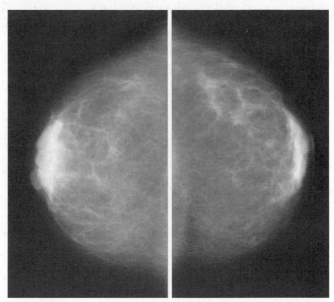

CC

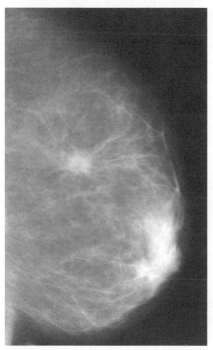

ML

1. Describe the subtle mammographic finding.

2. Does the addition of the straight lateral view help?

3. Give a differential diagnosis for the mammographic finding.

4. Explain the subtly of the findings based on the expected histologic tumor type.

Invasive Lobular Cancer

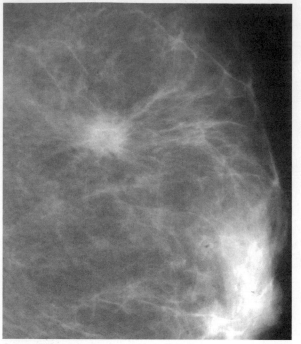

Cropped ML view

1. There is a subtle focal asymmetry in the upper outer right breast. There is a suggestion of slight architectural distortion.

2. The straight lateral view better demonstrates an area of architectural distortion in the upper right breast.

3. The differential diagnosis includes invasive lobular carcinoma and, less likely, invasive ductal carcinoma or a radial scar. Of course, a clinical history must be taken to exclude that the area of distortion is due to prior surgery.

4. The visualization of architectural distortion seen best in one plane suggests the histologic finding of invasive lobular carcinoma.

References

Le Gal M, Ollivier L, Asselain B, Meunier M, Laurent M, Vielh P, Neuenschwander S: Mammographic features of 455 invasive lobular carcinomas, *Radiology* 185:705–708, 1992.

Samardar P, Shaw de Paredes E, Grimes MM, Wilson JD: Focal asymmetric densities seen at mammography: US and pathologic correlation, *RadioGraphics* 22: 19–33, 2002.

Cross-Reference

Ikeda, *Breast Imaging: THE REQUISITES*, p 97.

Comment

This is an example of a subtle area of distortion due to invasive lobular carcinoma that is most evident on the straight lateral or medial lateral 90° (ML) view. On the initial MLO and CC views, there is a suggestion of a focal asymmetry in the upper outer right breast, but no definite mass is seen and the asymmetry has a mixed density, including areas of fat. To further evaluate the asymmetry, a spot compression view would be performed and a ML view. The distortion in this case was best seen in the ML view.

Invasive lobular carcinoma (ILC) accounts for approximately 10% of all breast cancers and is characterized microscopically by linear invasive columns of cells that are loosely dispersed. This is in contrast to the mammographic appearance of invasive ductal carcinoma, which is more typically seen as a high-density, discrete, and irregular mass. ILC frequently invades normal tissues without evoking the very severe desmoplastic response that usually accompanies infiltrating ductal carcinomas. Therefore, the linear arrangement of the cells of infiltrating lobular carcinoma often preserves the architecture of the ducts and the infiltration extends between fat lobules. These histologic features tend to produce a more subtle mammographic finding that is seen in the more common infiltrating ductal carcinoma.

Mammographically, there is usually no definite mass or a cluster of microcalcifications associated with infiltrating lobular carcinoma. Therefore, ILC in general presents at a larger size than invasive ductal carcinoma. The most common mammographic finding includes vague asymmetries, poorly defined opacities, or architectural distortions. On clinical presentation, there may be only thickening or asymmetry on breast exam. Often, there is no mammographic finding in very dense breasts in which there is not significant architectural distortion. Sonographically, the most common appearance is a heterogeneous hypoechoic mass with angular ill-defined margins and posterior shadowing. The architectural distortion, however, may be subtle, causing shadowing without a discrete mass seen. ILC has a higher incidence of being multicentric or bilateral than invasive ductal carcinoma. Some authors suggest that the bilaterality is approximately 10–15%. Therefore, imaging evaluation of the contralateral breast is imperative.

Notes

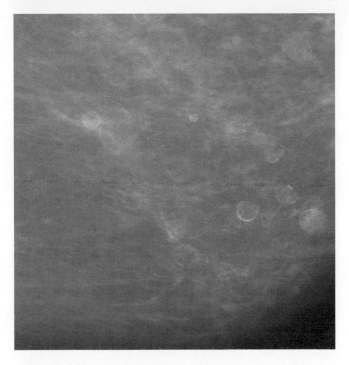

1. Describe findings on the magnification view above.

2. What is the most likely cause of these findings?

3. Is any further workup needed?

4. What diagnosis should be considered if these findings are bilateral and diffuse?

Oil Cysts

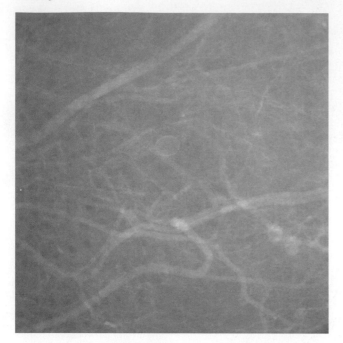

1. There are multiple well-circumscribed masses that have lucent fat density centers. Some of the small masses are beginning to calcify in their periphery.

2. These are oil cysts, and they are most likely due to some form of trauma.

3. No further evaluation is needed—BI-RADS category 2: benign.

4. Steatocystoma multiplex

References
American College of Radiology: *Illustrated BI-RADS*, ed 4, Reston, VA, 2004, American College of Radiology, pp 76–81.

Sickles EA: Breast calcifications: Mammographic evaluation, *Radiology* 160:289–293, 1986.

Cross-Reference
Ikeda, *Breast Imaging: THE REQUISITES*, pp 73, 122.

Comment
Calcifications with lucent centers are one of the classic types of benign calcifications. This subgroup of benign calcifications occurs in various conditions. Very thin-rimmed calcifications are called eggshell calcifications and are seen associated with oil cysts or fat necrosis. Small-caliber, lucent-centered calcifications with a relatively thick wall may be seen in the skin or can form around debris in a duct.

The small round masses with lucent centers seen in this case are due to benign oil cysts. Mammographically, these masses are well circumscribed and appear "encapsulated." The central lucency is from liquefied fat. Over time, the thin surrounding capsules may calcify, as in this case. Clinically, patients may be asymptomatic, or occasionally they may present with an area of palpable concern that is often small, superficial, and palpable. When ultrasound is performed, round or oval masses are seen that are usually hypoechoic or anechoic, but sometimes there may be mixed echoes internally due to the fat. In addition, if there is a sharp capsule or early rim calcifications, posterior acoustic shadowing may be seen on ultrasound.

Multiple bilateral oil cysts may be due to steatocystoma multiplex. In this rare autosomal disorder, which is usually seen in males, multiple cutaneous intradermal cysts are present, usually on the upper extremity and trunk. Patients may present with palpable freely mobile small superficial nodules that may become inflamed. There is no malignant potential.

Notes

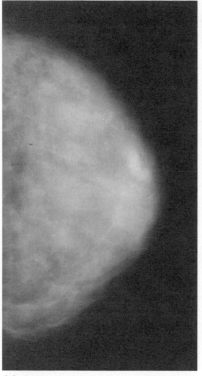

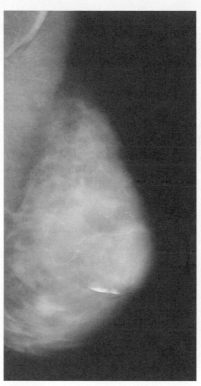

CC view   ML view

1. Describe the mammographic findings.
2. What is the most likely diagnosis?
3. What BI-RADS category is appropriate?
4. What is the anatomic site of origin of this type of calcification?

Milk of Calcium

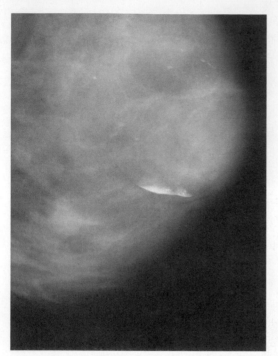

1. There is a suggestion of a focal asymmetry associated with amorphous calcifications on the two views. The straight lateral view shows a "meniscus" or "teacup" calcification.

2. This is consistent with milk of calcium in a macrocyst.

3. BI-RADS category 2: benign.

4. Micro- and macrocysts tend to occur in the acini of the lobule.

References

Sickles EA: Milk of calcium with tiny benign breast cysts, *Radiology* 141:655–658, 1981.
Sickles EA: Breast calcifications: Mammographic evaluation, *Radiology* 160:289–293, 1986.

Cross-Reference

Ikeda, *Breast Imaging: THE REQUISITES*, p 75.

Comment

There is a suggestion of focal asymmetry or possibly a mass in the anterior portion of the breast. The calcifications associated with a focal asymmetry are amorphous or smudgy on the cranial caudal view. The orthogonal, 90° lateral view confirms the benign nature of the calcifications and the focal asymmetry. The mass is a macrocyst and there is dependent "milk of calcium" layering in the cyst. No further evaluation is needed. The fact that there is milk of calcium in suspension in the macrocyst confirms the benign nature. The pathoneumonic appearance of a meniscus or teacup of dependent calcifications on the straight lateral view confirms a benign diagnosis and no further imaging is necessary. Occasionally, the calcifications are not in solution but may be small, round concretions that appear like pearls in a sac, best seen on the straight lateral view. Histologically, these micro- or macrocysts form in dilated acini of the lobule or in a dilated portion of a terminal duct.

Notes

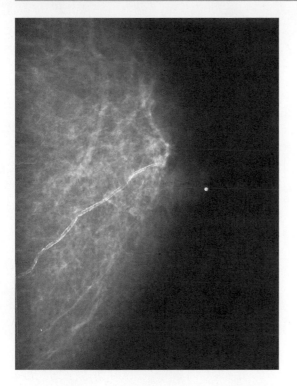

1. What type of calcifications is represented here?
2. What may these calcifications indicate?
3. Is any follow-up needed?
4. Are the calcifications indicative of increased breast cancer risk?

Vascular Calcifications

1. Vascular calcifications.

2. Diabetes mellitus and connective tissue diseases may predispose a patient to forming vascular calcifications at a young age. Arteriosclerosis also occurs as an aging process.

3. No mammographic follow-up is needed. The patient may consider being evaluated for arteriosclerosis, or more clinical information regarding medical history may be obtained.

4. No.

References

Moshyedi AC, Puthawala AH, Kurland RJ, O'Leary DH: Breast arterial calcification: Association with coronary artery disease, *Radiology* 194:181–183, 1995.

Van Noord PA, Beijerinck D, Kemmerenen JM, Graaf Y: Mammograms may convey more than breast cancer risk: Breast arterial calcification and arterio-sclerotic related diseases in women of the DOM cohort, *Eur J Cancer Prev* 5:483–487, 1996.

Cross-Reference

Ikeda, *Breast Imaging: THE REQUISITES*, p 81.

Comment

This patient is in her thirties. She is undergoing routine screening mammography because her mother was diagnosed with breast cancer at age 34. Calcifications were noted on her mammogram. These vascular calcifications may be mentioned in the mammogram report, and mention made of possible increased risk of cardiac disease.

Typically, vascular calcifications do not cause difficulty in diagnosis. Characteristically, they are seen as parallel lines of calcification, often with amorphous calcification within the parallel lines, indicating the vessel wall en face. This is much more commonly seen in patients older than 60 years of age. These typical calcifications need no further workup.

The vascular calcifications seen on mammography are in the media of the smaller vessel walls, the arterioles, and not in the intima of the wall, as is seen in large arteries. The risk of the development of this calcification is increased in diabetes and chronic renal failure, and there may be an increased risk factor for coronary artery disease. The calcifications are not related to breast disease.

Notes

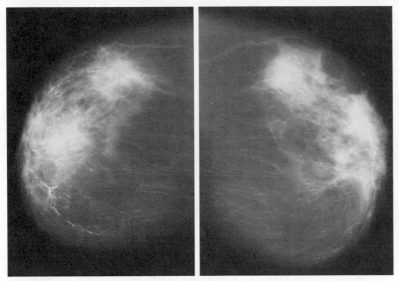

CC views

1. The baseline mammogram in this 68-year-old shows diffuse bilateral calcifications. What is the differential diagnosis?

2. Are any additional mammographic images needed?

3. What are the histologic findings?

4. What recommendations for intervention and/or follow-up are given? Please give a BI-RADS category.

Secretory Calcifications

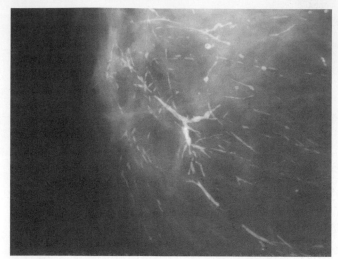

Left mag

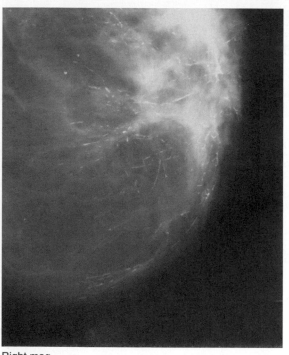

Right mag

1. The calcifications in this case are coarse and linear, consistent with benign secretory disease or plasma cell mastitis.

2. In this case, no additional imaging is needed. However, if there were faint indeterminate calcifications, magnification views would be necessary.

3. Histologically, there are dilated ducts with periductal inflammation.

4. Intervention is unnecessary. BI-RADS category 2: benign. Routine follow-up.

References

Bassett LW, Jackson VP, Jahan R, Fu YS, Gold RH: *Diagnosis of Diseases of the Breast*, Philadelphia, 1997, Saunders.

Cardenosa G: *The Core Curriculum: Breast Imaging*, Baltimore, 2004, Lippincott Williams & Wilkins.

Cross-Reference

Ikeda, *Breast Imaging: THE REQUISITES*, pp 77–79.

Comment

The mammogram reveals bilateral diffuse calcifications in a ductal distribution. The calcifications are dense, thick, and rodlike. Some actually show branching, and others are tubular with a lucent center. The large rod-like calcifications have tapered ends or cigar shapes. There are also periductal calcifications forming around dilated debris-filled ducts. These calcifications look like long hollow tubes. Inspection of the calcifications shows that the size and smooth margins of the tapering calcifications are much larger than the more irregular pleomorphic calcifications of DCIS. These calcifications are typical of those seen in benign secretory disease or plasma cell mastitis and duct ectasia.

Histologically, the dilated ducts are thick walled and contain thick creamy debris and foam cells. The process is often bilateral and diffuse but may occasionally be unilateral and focal. Focal changes may be more difficult to differentiate from comedo ductal carcinoma *in situ*. Magnification views may be helpful in focal cases to look for the typical periductal calcifications with lucent centers and smooth margins vs finer linear irregular calcifications of high-grade DCIS. No intervention is needed for a typical case of bilateral and diffuse plasma cell mastitis, as shown in this case. New, more focal and irregular calcifications, however, may require biopsy to exclude malignancy.

Notes

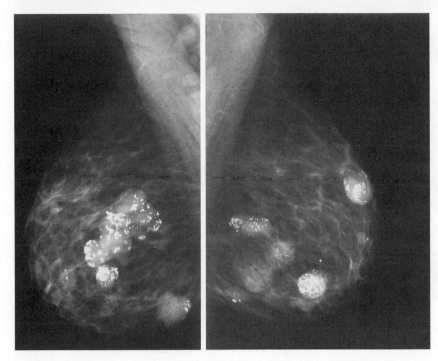

1. The patient is asymptomatic and both breasts have a similar appearance. What is the most likely diagnosis?

2. Histologically, what are the popcorn calcifications due to?

3. What is the BI-RADS category?

4. How often are these masses multiple or bilateral?

Calcified Fibroadenomas

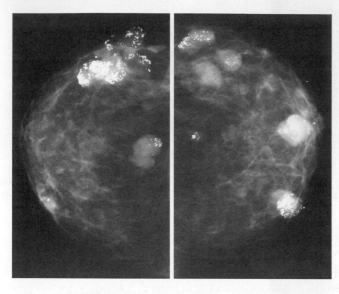

1. Multiple bilateral fibroadenomas.

2. Calcifications occur due to involution of the benign fibroadenomas.

3. BI-RADS category 2: benign, no evidence of malignancy.

4. Approximately 15–20%.

Reference

Bassett LW, Jackson VP, Jahan R, Fu YS, Gold RH: *Diagnosis of Diseases of the Breast*, Philadelphia, 1997, Saunders, p 386.

Cross-Reference

Ikeda, *Breast Imaging: THE REQUISITES*, pp 79–80.

Comment

This asymptomatic patient presented for screening mammography with bilateral masses that are associated with coarse, popcorn calcifications, some of which are peripheral. This postmenopausal woman has a very typical appearance of involuting fibroadenomas. No further evaluation is needed. Of course, close scrutiny of the mammogram is necessary to ensure that there are no other findings that are of concern.

Fibroadenomas are the most common solid mass in women. Mammographically, they are frequently well-circumscribed oval masses, and on sonography they are often well-circumscribed, hypoechoic masses with a thin echogenic rim and a wider than tall orientation. Coarse popcorn-type calcifications occur with involution of these masses usually after menopause. The calcifications frequently begin at the periphery of the mass and move toward the center, and often the calcifications may completely replace the mass mammographically. In this case, no further evaluation is needed and a BI-RADS category 2, benign, is adequate. Routine follow-up is sufficient.

Notes

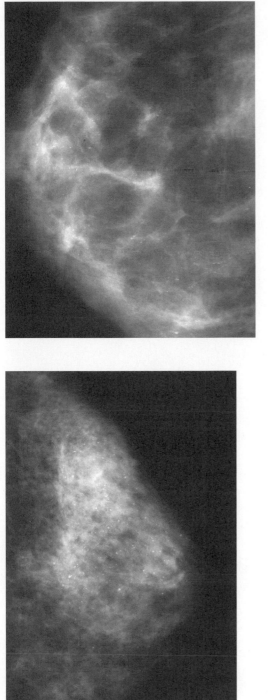

1. What characterizes the calcifications in these three different patients?

2. Are the calcifications typically benign?

3. Can these calcifications be followed, or is biopsy indicated? BI-RADS?

4. How can DCIS be distinguished from these benign-type calcifications?

Diffuse Calcifications

1. There are many calcifications scattered throughout the breasts.

2. The calcifications are punctate, without suspicious clustering, and are typically benign.

3. These calcifications can be followed with annual mammography. BI-RADS 2.

4. To distinguish DCIS, look for linear alignment, branching forms, tight clusters, and pleomorphism.

Reference

Sickles EA: Breast calcifications: Mammographic evaluation, *Radiology* 160:289–293, 1986.

Cross-Reference

Ikeda, *Breast Imaging: THE REQUISITES*, p 70.

Comment

Features of calcifications that must be assessed during the interpretation of the mammogram include the morphology of the calcifications and their distribution. In these examples, the calcifications are punctate, a clearly benign morphology. The distribution is diffuse, scattered throughout the breast. A search must be made for suspicious forms, such as clustered, branching forms, which may be present within the scattered benign forms. Viewing the mammogram with a magnifying lens should help one decide whether the patient needs to return for additional mammographic views. Comparison with prior films is also extremely helpful. If prior films are not available, magnification views can be performed if you are in doubt as to the nature of the calcifications. Magnification views are performed in two projections, CC and 90° true lateral. The 90° lateral view is used instead of MLO to more clearly see layering of milk of calcium if it is present.

Notes

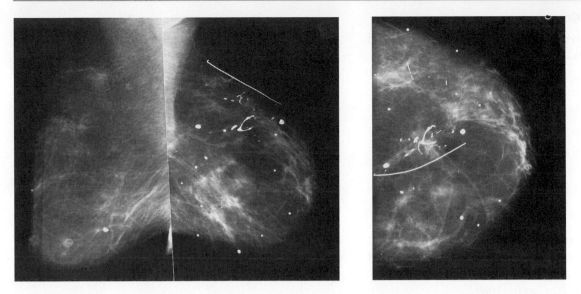

1. This elderly woman had a benign surgical biopsy many years ago. How can you tell from the images?

2. What do the curvilinear calcifications represent?

3. Is this type of calcification common?

4. Is there a differential diagnosis?

CASE 38

Suture Calcification

1. She has thick curvilinear calcifications at the surgical site. The scar on the skin is marked with a metal marker.

2. She has calcification of suture material placed by the surgeon at the time of biopsy.

3. It is unusual to see suture calcification.

4. When the suture calcification is linear, it can be mistaken for secretory-type calcifications, also possibly confused with intraductal cancer.

Reference

Davis SP, Stomper PC, Weidner N, Meyer JE: Suture calcification mimicking recurrence in the irradiated breast: A potential pitfall in mammographic evaluation, *Radiology* 172:247–248, 1989.

Cross-Reference

Ikeda, *Breast Imaging: THE REQUISITES*, pp 314–315.

Comment

Calcification in suture material represents an artifact in the patient—a man-made structure that causes an abnormal density in the breast. Most suture material is invisible on mammography, and rarely does the material calcify. However, calcium can be deposited on suture material, and when it is seen, it is typically linear or tubular in shape. If a knot is seen in the calcified suture, there will be no doubt of the diagnosis of suture calcifications. Calcification may develop in catgut suture material, which contains dead collagen. The calcifications in suture may mimic recurrent disease at the lumpectomy site. Magnification views should be performed if there is any question about the origin of the calcifications.

The scar on the patient's skin can be marked with a metal marker, indicating the site of prior surgery. The suture calcifications should be seen in the vicinity of the scar.

Notes

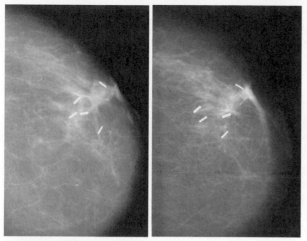

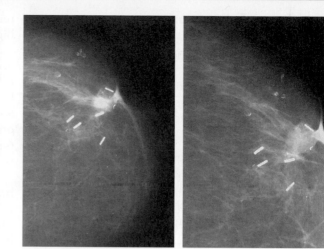

1 year post XRT

18 months post XRT

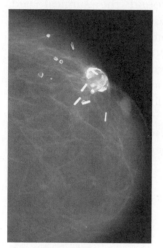

3 years post XRT

1. This patient has had a lumpectomy for ductal carcinoma *in situ*. What initial follow-up is recommended after the lumpectomy?

2. What is recommended for the patient after the completion of radiation therapy and why?

3. What are the expected benign changes following breast conservation and radiation therapy?

4. How common are recurrences?

Postlumpectomy Fat Necrosis

1. In patients who have had breast conservation therapy and have had mammographically detected calcifications associated with their cancers, a mammogram with magnification views is recommended to assess for residual calcifications after lumpectomy and prior to radiation.

2. Follow-up recommendations are somewhat controversial, but most centers recommend at least an annual bilateral diagnostic mammogram at the completion of radiation therapy. Other centers follow patients every 6 months for 2 years after completion of radiation therapy.

3. Early mammographic changes after lumpectomy and radiation are increased density in the surgical bed associated with architectural distortion. There may also be skin and trabecular thickening from the radiation therapy. Over time, coarse peripheral calcifications around a central lucency often develop in the surgical bed from fat necrosis.

4. Recurrence occurs at a rate of approximately 1% per year, with early recurrences near the surgical bed (possibly due to residual disease). In later years, the development of a second primary cancer is more common than the presence of residual cancer or actual recurrence of the original cancer.

References

Giess CS, Keating DM, Osborne MP, Rosenblatt R: Local tumor recurrence following breast-conservation therapy: Correlation of histopathologic findings with detection method and mammographic findings, *Radiology* 212:829–835, 1999.

Giess CS, Keating DM, Osborne MP, Mester J, Rosenblatt R: Comparison of rate of development and rate of change for benign and malignant breast calcifications at the lumpectomy bed, *Am J Roentgenol* 175:789–793, 2000.

Cross-Reference

Ikeda, *Breast Imaging: THE REQUISITES*, p 240.

Comment

The aim of breast conservation is to locally control breast cancer and, with clear surgical margins, to minimize the recurrence of the original disease. In cancers that contain calcifications as part of the mammographic presentation, postsurgical imaging is needed to ensure all the "malignant" calcifications have been removed. The imaging, performed in orthogonal planes with magnification, should be done after the lumpectomy and prior to the initiation of radiation therapy. Any remaining suspicious calcifications correlate with a higher incidence of residual disease and recurrence.

Mammographic changes after lumpectomy and radiation are variable, and although yearly diagnostic imaging follow-up is the norm, often short-term follow-up may be necessary to ensure the evolving changes are benign. Some sites will follow these patients with either unilateral (the radiated breast) or bilateral mammograms at 6-month intervals for up to 2 years after the completion of radiation therapy.

Initially, there is often edema and thickening of the breasts after radiation therapy, and the distorted surgical bed may be dense due to a seroma or hematoma. The density and size of the surgical bed should decrease during the first 2 years, and frequently there are characteristic changes of fat necrosis with oil cyst formation and the development of coarse, dystrophic, and often peripheral calcifications around the surgical bed. However, the early calcifications of fat necrosis may be somewhat irregular or pleomorphic and concerning. Close follow-up of these dystrophic calcifications with short-term follow-up and magnification views is needed to ensure that the calcifications do indeed evolve into classic coarse peripheral calcifications rather than calcifications due to residual disease. Early recurrence or the detection of residual disease tends to occur at or close to the lumpectomy site. If there is concern for residual disease or recurrence, biopsy is necessary.

Notes

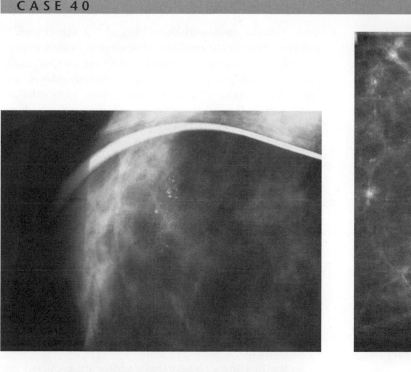
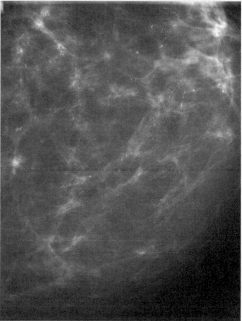
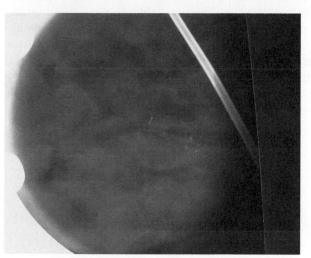

1. What is the abnormal finding in each of these three different patients? What is the BI-RADS code when seen on a screening mammogram?

2. What is the next step in the workup?

3. What are the three options after the mammographic workup?

4. Is any additional imaging (e.g., ultrasound or MRI) needed?

Suspicious Calcifications

1. There are microcalcifications in the breast (BI-RADS 0).

2. Magnification views are the next step.

3. After the magnification views are performed, one needs to decide if the calcifications can be followed in 6 months (BI-RADS 3), biopsied with the needle core technique, or surgically excised (BI-RADS 4).

4. Ultrasound and MRI have limited usefulness for evaluating suspicious microcalcifications. Calcifications may be missed on ultrasound, unless there is an associated mass. MRI is not as sensitive for DCIS as it is for invasive malignancy.

References

Berg WA, Arnoldus CL, Teferra E, Bhargavan M: Biopsy of amorphous breast calcifications: Pathologic outcome and yield at stereotactic biopsy, *Radiology* 221:495–503, 2001.

Dershaw DD, Abramson A, Kinne DW: Ductal carcinoma *in situ*: Mammographic findings and clinical implications, *Radiology* 170:411–415, 1989.

Sickles EA: Breast calcifications: Mammographic evaluation, *Radiology* 160:289–293, 1986.

Cross-Reference

Ikeda, *Breast Imaging: THE REQUISITES*, p 62.

Comment

In evaluating calcifications, magnification views are essential. If performed with a proper technique, the views will provide needed information to help determine whether the calcifications are more likely to be benign or malignant. If microcalcifications are seen on a conventional screening mammogram, it is best to recall the patient for additional magnification views rather than to try to make a diagnosis on the standard screening images.

Magnification views are often performed in the 90° lateral view to check for layering. If the calcifications layer on this view, they can be reliably characterized as benign, needing no further evaluation.

Determining benign from suspicious calcifications is a step-by-step process. The first step is to analyze the magnification views and determine if the calcifications fall into any of the definitely benign categories (round, eggshell, coarse linear, and popcorn).

The next step is to decide if the calcifications are suspicious for malignancy. Suspicious calcifications are pleomorphic and may have irregular margins or broken glass shapes. Calcifications of DCIS form inside the duct, making casts and branching along the course of the duct. Calcifications that are neither definitely benign nor suspicious may be termed *indeterminate for malignancy*. In this category are coarse, heterogenous, and amorphous forms, which are faint, small, hazy calcifications. If their distribution is linear or segmental, which are more suggestive of malignancy, biopsy is recommended.

The distribution of the calcifications as well as the individual morphology are important. Distribution is categorized as follows (in order of increasing level of suspicion):

1. Diffuse, which is distributed throughout most of the breast
2. Regional, distributed in an area at least 2 cm of the breast, not in ductal distribution
3. Grouped or clustered (at least five calcifications in less than 1 cc of tissue)
4. Linear, forms suggestive of ducts
5. Segmental, distributed in a lobe or segment of the breast, suspicious for involving a duct and its branches

In the first image, the calcifications are grouped and are amorphous and pleomorphic. In the second image, there are many fine linear calcifications. In the third image, a branching form is seen. Stereotactic biopsy was performed in all three patients, and these calcifications all represent DCIS.

Notes

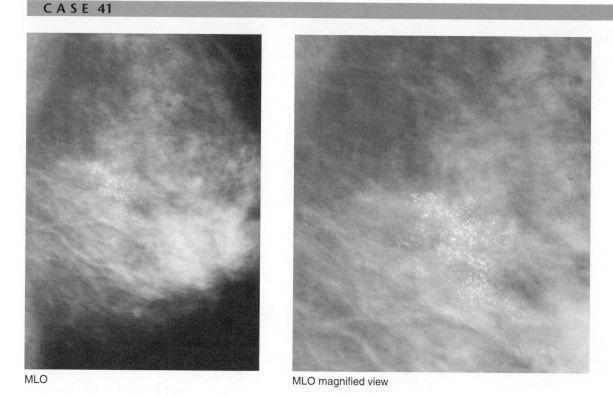

MLO

MLO magnified view

1. Describe the calcifications seen on this diagnostic mammogram. What BI-RADS category should be given?

2. What is the most likely histology for these calcifications?

3. What percentage of mammographically detected breast malignancies are DCIS?

4. How well does mammography estimate the extent of disease?

DCIS—Comedo Carcinoma

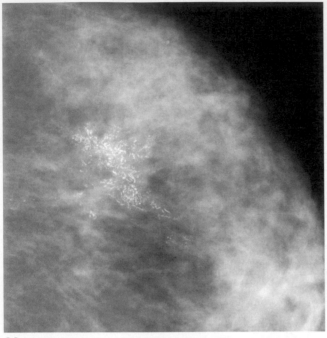

CC mag

1. The mammogram shows linear branching pleomorphic calcifications, which are also forming casts of the ductal system. The appearance is highly suspicious for DCIS. BI-RADS category 5: highly suspicious.

2. The appearance of these casting calcifications is highly suspicious for high-grade comedo carcinoma, a subtype of DCIS.

3. Approximately 30% of cancers detected mammographically are due to DCIS.

4. In high-grade comedo carcinoma, the calcifications tend to occur discretely within the cancer; therefore, mammographic measurements provide an accurate estimate of disease extent. This is not true for all forms of breast cancer.

References

Bassett LW, Liu HS, Giuliano A, Gold RH: Prevalence of carcinoma in palpable versus impalpable mammographically detected lesions, *Am J Roentgenol* 157: 21–24, 1991.

Bassett LW, Jackson VP, Jahan R, Fu YS, Gold RH: *Diagnosis of Diseases of the Breast*, Philadelphia, 1997, Saunders, pp 446–448.

Cross-Reference

Ikeda, *Breast Imaging: THE REQUISTES*, pp 62–67.

Comment

These calcifications are the typical casting calcifications seen associated with the necrosis of high-grade comedo carcinoma, a subtype of DCIS. This tumor arises in the terminal ductal lobular unit and grows in the duct toward the nipple. Comedo carcinoma is a poorly differentiated form of DCIS that tends to have a continuous growth of tumor along the ductal system. Other subtypes of DCIS have a higher incidence of discontinuous or skip-type growth patterns. Because of the very coarse and pleomorphic calcifications, and the tendency for a continuous growth pattern, the linear branching calcifications seen on mammography often provide a fairly accurate estimate of lesion size. However, it is known that as the volume of DCIS increases, the chance of microinvasion increases as well. In particular, when the extent of disease seen mammographically is 2.5 cm or greater, the likelihood of microinvasion is high enough that many surgeons will perform lymph node dissection even though no invasion may be documented histologically.

The mammogram should be evaluated for multicentric and multifocal disease, and any suspicious areas of calcifications should be biopsied to document the extent of disease. A clinical presentation of this type of DCIS is asymptomatic in the majority of cases. Rarely, a patient may present with a palpable mass, but in these cases, there is a higher likelihood of associated invasive carcinoma. Comedo carcinoma is associated with a higher rate of recurrence and other subtypes of DCIS. This is due to the high nuclear grade and the radio resistance of the tumor.

Notes

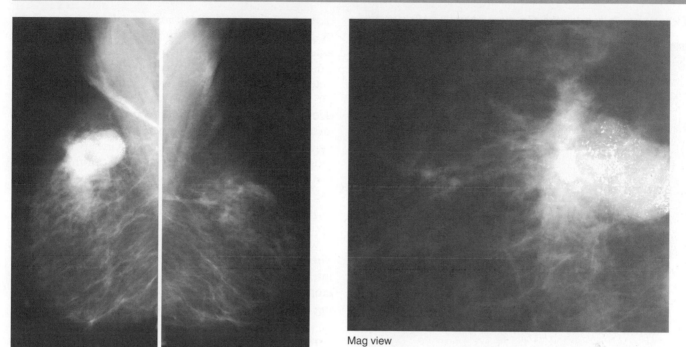

Mag view

MLOs

1. Describe the mammographic findings in this case.

2. What is the significance of the calcifications in the lesion?

3. How should this lesion be localized for surgical excision if breast conservation is chosen?

4. Why is giving measurements of the size of the lesion important for the referring physician or surgeon?

Extensive Intraductal Component

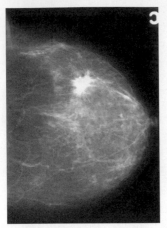

Another patient

1. Mammographically, there is a highly suspicious spiculated mass with associated pleomorphic calcifications.

2. The calcifications are concerning for a extensive intraductal component (EIC) of this tumor.

3. Surgically, it is important if breast conservation is performed to excise not only the spiculated mass but also the calcifications extending in a ductal distribution from the mass.

4. Giving the measurements of the extent of disease is very important. Not only does this description of the extent of disease help determine whether breast conservation or mastectomy is needed but also the description of the highly pleomorphic calcifications may relate to the prognosis of the patient.

Reference

Stomper PC, Connolly JL: Mammographic features predicting an extensive intraductal component in early stage infiltrating ductal carcinoma, *Am J Roentgenol* 158:269–272, 1992.

Cross-Reference

Ikeda, *Breast Imaging: THE REQUISITES*, p 92.

Comment

The mammographic findings here are almost pathognemonic for a invasive ductal carcinoma with an extensive area of associated intraductal carcinoma. These tumors, which are described as having an EIC, have a worse prognosis and a higher incidence of local recurrence after breast conservation surgery and radiation therapy. This is most likely related to the EIC and incomplete resection of the lesion. It is very important to do a careful mammographic evaluation so the extent of the calcifications is clearly described. Magnification views of the surrounding tissue extending anteriorly toward the nipple may often reveal additional clusters of suspicious calcifications. A core biopsy will determine that this is an invasive ductal carcinoma, but for a complete surgical excision if breast conservation is deemed possible, the entire extent of the suspicious area must be localized with bracketing needles. This is performed with needles and guidewires placed at the most posterior and most anterior aspect of the lesion so that any visible intraductal disease is also resected with the invasive component.

A postlumpectomy mammogram is necessary if breast conservation is desired to ensure that the entire extent of calcifications have been removed surgically. These lesions frequently have "skip" involvement of the intraductal component, and therefore it is very important to try to guide the surgeons with an excellent imaging workup and localization at surgery.

Notes

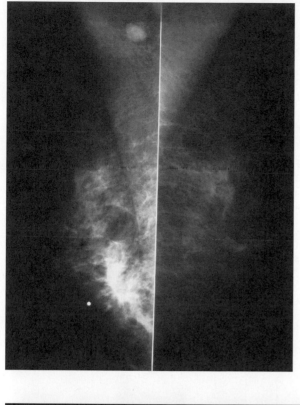

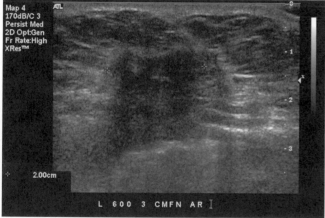

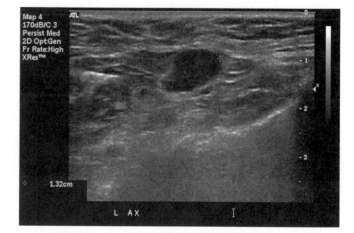

1. What is the abnormality on this mammogram?

2. Is there any abnormality in the axilla?

3. What is the next diagnostic step in the workup?

4. Does needle biopsy of the axillary lesion help in the workup?

Suspicious Mass and Axillary Node

1. There is a dense, spiculated, suspicious mass in the lower left breast.

2. There is an enlarged, dense node in the axilla.

3. Ultrasound can be used next for several reasons:
   (i) to evaluate the mammographic mass,
   (ii) to evaluate for any additional masses, and
   (iii) to evaluate the axillary node.

4. Needle biopsy of the abnormal node may obviate the need for sentinel node biopsy if the cytology shows metastatic disease.

References

Feu J, Tresserra F, Fabregas R, Navarro B, Grases PJ, Suris JC, Fernandez-Cid A, Alegret X: Metastatic breast carcinoma in axillary lymph nodes: In vitro US detection, *Radiology* 205(3):831–835, 1997.

Yang WT, Chang J, Metreweli C: Patients with breast cancer: Differences in color Doppler flow and gray-scale US features of benign and malignant axillary lymph nodes, *Radiology* 215:568–573, 2000.

Cross-Reference

Ikeda, *Breast Imaging: THE REQUISITES*, p 303.

Comment

In this patient, there is a suspicious mass in the lower aspect of the left breast. The workup needs to focus on three things:

1. The ultrasound appearance of the suspicious tumor. Ultrasound can be used to guide the needle core biopsy and confirm the malignant appearance of the mammographic finding.

2. Checking for multicentric and multifocal tumors, which may be adjacent to the original tumor, between the original tumor and the nipple, or in a separate quadrant of the breast.

3. Checking the axilla for abnormal nodes. If an enlarged, dense node is seen in the axilla on the mammogram, this should be confirmed on ultrasound. Sometimes the apparently abnormal node has a normal appearance on ultrasound.

The normal lymph node should have a characteristic appearance on ultrasound. There is an echogenic fatty central hilus, which is variable in size. There is a concentric hypoechoic cortex surrounding the hilus.

Abnormal nodes have evidence of infiltration into the cortex, so the cortex is asymmetric, bulging on one side, causing the fatty hilus to become eccentric. The infiltration gradually effaces the hilus and then obliterates it. As the node becomes infiltrated, it changes from oval to rounded. The more severely involved node is hypoechoic and may even appear cystic or anechoic. Cysts do not occur in the axilla, as a rule, and should not be in your differential diagnosis of a hypoic mass in the axilla. Color-flow Doppler can be used to demonstrate the presence of blood flow in a hypoechoic mass. The presence of blood flow within the mass indicates that the mass is solid, not a cyst.

Lymph nodes may have a normal appearance and may still harbor metastatic cells. The use of fine-needle aspiration biopsy of axillary lymph nodes can give important information to the surgeon prior to definitive surgery.

If the needle aspirate shows malignant cells, the patient may undergo an axillary dissection instead of sentinel node biopsy.

Notes

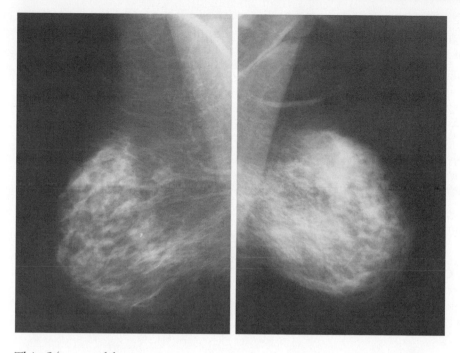

This 54-year-old woman presents with a heavy or thickened right breast with minimal tenderness on exam.

1. Describe the mammographic findings.
2. What is the differential diagnosis for a unilateral diffuse breast change?
3. Is ultrasound useful in determining the etiology of this condition?
4. What is the next diagnostic procedure?

Inflammatory Carcinoma

1. Mammographically, there is skin and trabecular thickening and a global asymmetry of the breast.

2. The differential diagnosis includes inflammatory carcinoma, infectious mastitis, diffuse invasive lobular carcinoma, or lymphomatous involvement of the breast. The clinical presentation is most consistent with inflammatory carcinoma.

3. Ultrasound is often nonspecific; however, it may be helpful in localizing a discrete mass for percutaneous biopsy.

4. A biopsy is needed that includes the dermis to help differentiate between benign and malignant etiologies.

Reference

Kushwaha AC, Whitman GJ, Stelling CB, Cristofanilli M, Buzdar AU: Primary inflammatory carcinoma of the breast: Retrospective review of mammographic findings, *Am J Roentgenol* 174(2):535–538, 2000.

Cross-Reference

Ikeda, *Breast Imaging: THE REQUISITES*, p 151.

Comment

The diagnosis of inflammatory carcinoma is made on clinical findings. Patients often describe a rapid onset of unilateral breast thickening, edema, and erythema but little pain. Conversely, although diffuse bacterial mastitis may present with somewhat similar clinical findings, there is usually significant tenderness and often a fever. A course of antibiotics may cause slight improvement in inflammatory carcinoma, but there should be significant improvement with antibiotics when there is bacterial mastitis. The definitive diagnosis of inflammatory carcinoma must be made by biopsy. Histologically, inflammatory carcinoma is most often due to a poorly differentiated invasive ductal carcinoma with tumor emboli in the dilated dermal lymphatics. There is often a lymphocytic reaction surrounding the large dilated vessels of the dermis. The clinical presentation, however, is not specific to invasive ductal carcinoma but may also be seen in invasive lobular.

Unilateral diffuse increased parenchymal densities are the most common mammographic findings of inflammatory carcinoma. Axillary adenopathy has been reported in 58% of these patients at presentation. Both adenopathy and global involvement may be seen with diffuse invasive lobular carcinoma and lymphomatus involvement of the breast, and the diagnosis again must be made by biopsy. Ultrasound may be helpful to localize a specific mass to guide biopsy. However, diffuse skin thickening and dilated lymphatics may make penetrating the breast with ultrasound difficult. Ultrasound may also be used to localize suspicious nodes for biopsy. Similarly, MRI may reveal focal areas of suspicious enhancement to guide biopsies.

Notes

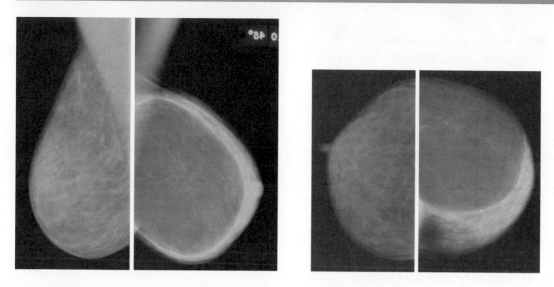

1. What additional studies, if any, are needed in this 60-year-old woman with this baseline screening mammogram?

2. What is this mass?

3. What is the BI-RADS assessment category and follow-up recommendation for this patient?

4. If this mass was palpable, would the recommendation for follow-up differ?

Lipoma

1. The fat density mass in the breast requires no additional imaging.

2. This is a lipoma.

3. This is a BI-RADS category 2 benign lesion. Routine follow-up is recommended.

4. Correlation with physical exam is recommended, but this mass requires no additional imaging. Lipomas may occasionally be palpable but correspond in size to the mass seen mammographically.

References

Lanng C, Eriksen BO, Hoffmann J: Lipoma of the breast: A diagnostic dilemma, *Breast* 13(5):408–411, 2004.

Rodriguez LF, Shuster BA, Milliken RG: Giant lipoma of the breast, *Br J Plastic Surg* 50(4):263–265, 1997.

Cross-Reference

Ikeda, *Breast Imaging: THE REQUISTES*, p 122.

Comment

The mammogram reveals a large, totally lucent, well-circumscribed mass with a thin fibrous capsule consistent with a benign lipoma. No further imaging evaluation is needed and certainly no biopsy is indicated. This is a category 2 benign lesion and there is only a short differential diagnosis, including fibroadenolipoma (hamartoma) or fibrolipoma (containing more fibrous tissue).

Lipomas are usually asymptomatic, as in this case, but may present as a mobile palpable mass. When there is a palpable mass, the size of the mass must be correlated with the size of the mammographic area of lucency. If there is a discordance, an ultrasound must be performed to ensure that there is no other mass that may be of concern. If the workup is for a woman younger than 30 years old, ultrasound may have been the initial study performed. In that case, a well-circumscribed mass with homogeneous hypoechoic-to-hyperechoic echotecture relative to the surrounding subcutaneous fat would be seen. Occasionally, lipomas may have the benign calcifications of fat necrosis. Histologically, the mass is composed of mature adipose cells surrounded by a thin capsule.

Notes

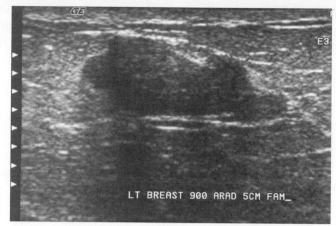

US

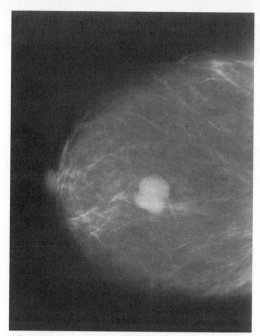

CC view

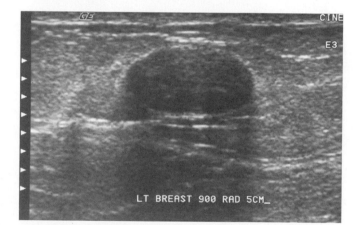

1. This 43-year-old woman presents with a nonpalpable mass in the right breast. Describe the mammographic findings.

2. Describe the ultrasound findings.

3. What is the most likely diagnosis?

4. What is the specificity of the ultrasound findings?

Macrolobulated Fibroadenoma

1. There is a lobulated, well-circumscribed, high-density mass in the center of the breast on this single image.

2. Ultrasound shows a macrolobulated homogeneously hypoechoic solid mass with a thin echogenic margin that is wider than tall.

3. Fibroadenoma.

4. Greater than 95% specificity.

References

Stavros AT, Thickman D, Rapp CL, Dennis MA, Parker SH, Sisney GA: Solid breast nodules: Use of sonography to distinguish between benign and malignant lesions, *Radiology* 196:123–134, 1995.

Stavros AT: *Breast Ultrasound*, Philadelphia, 2004, Lippincott Williams & Wilkins.

Cross-Reference

Ikeda, *Breast Imaging: THE REQUISITES*, p 110.

Comment

The mammogram shows a lobulated mass that could be due to either a complex cyst or a solid mass. Ultrasound in the radial and antiradial projections shows a macrolobulated mass that is wider than tall and has a thin echogenic margin. According to the Stavros criteria used to evaluate nonpalpable solid breast masses, the specificity of these findings is greater than 95% and the lesion most likely represents a benign fibroadenoma.

In 1995, Stavros described ultrasound criteria to evaluate nonpalpable solid breast masses. Benign ultrasound characteristics include macrolobulation, ovoid shape and a wider than tall orientation, and an echogenic rim with sharp anterior and posterior margins. Suspicious ultrasound characteristics according to Stavros include irregular or spiculated margins, duct extension, angular shape, a more taller than wide or vertical orientation, and marked posterior acoustic shadowing. According to his criteria, a mass should be considered suspicious if any of the malignant characteristics are seen.

The specificity of the very benign ultrasound findings in a solid mass, as in this case, is quite high. However, this mass is large, and if it is new, palpable, or rapidly growing, a biopsy is usually recommended to ensure that this is indeed a benign fibroadenoma.

If this patient thinks that the mass has been stable for many years, or if there are other similar-appearing masses in this breast or the contralateral breast or a history of previously biopsied fibroadenomas, it may be appropriate to follow the mass closely rather than to biopsy. If biopsy is chosen, a core biopsy under ultrasound should be sufficient to prove that this is a benign fibroadenoma.

Notes

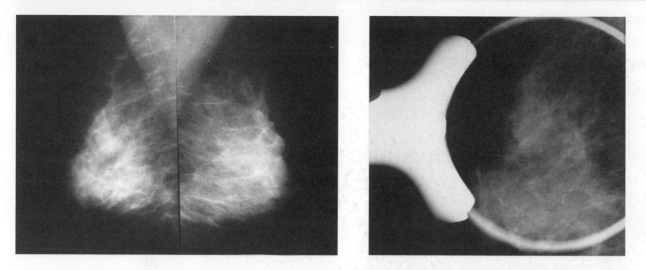

1. The glandular tissue is very dense. There is a partially obscured mass in the left upper breast. What is the next step in the workup?

2. Do the special views help in determining the nature of the finding?

3. Is the workup complete after the special views?

4. Is needle biopsy necessary?

Developing Mass with Obscured Margins—Cyst

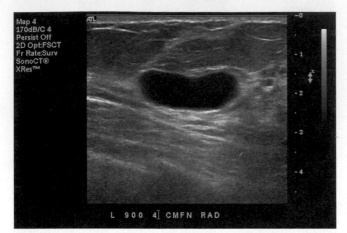

1. The next step is to perform spot compression views.

2. The spot compression views show persistence of the mass, with partially obscured margins.

3. The workup is incomplete. Ultrasound is indicated to determine the nature of the mass.

4. Needle sampling (aspiration) of the simple cyst is not necessary.

References

Berg WA: Cystic lesions of the breast: Sonographic–pathologic correlation, *Radiology* 227:183–191, 2003.

Rosner D, Blaird D: What ultrasonography can tell in breast masses that mammography and physical exam cannot, *J Surg Oncol* 28(4):308–313, 1985.

Cross-Reference

Ikeda, *Breast Imaging: THE REQUISITES*, p 122.

Comment

The mammogram has dense breast tissue, with a new round mass in the left upper outer breast. The margins of this mass are partially obscured. Spot compression views were performed and the margins are still partially obscured. By mammographic criteria, this cannot be confirmed to be a benign finding, so ultrasound is necessary.

Ultrasound of the mammographic finding confirms that it is a simple cyst. It has all five of the sonographic criteria to qualify as a simple cyst and is therefore definitely benign:

Anechoic
Well circumscribed
Thin, echogenic wall
Enhanced through transmission
Thin edge shadows

In the instance in which internal low-level echoes are seen inside the lesion, it is termed a *complicated cyst*. Occasionally, it may be difficult to distinguish between a complicated cyst with internal debris from a solid mass. Color-flow Doppler can be helpful in this situation: If there is color flow seen within the mass, it cannot be a complicated cyst but, rather, must be a solid mass. In rare cases, especially when the lesion is small, it may be necessary to attempt aspiration to prove it is a benign cyst. This simple procedure may be done under ultrasound guidance. In this particular case, no further evaluation is needed. Aspiration can be performed if the patient has pain or if the cyst is palpable and of concern either to the patient or to her physician.

Notes

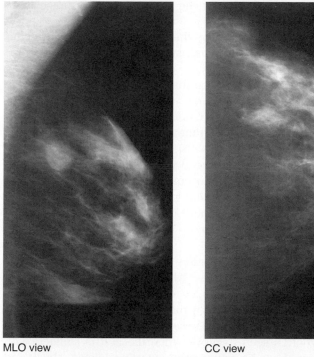

MLO view   CC view

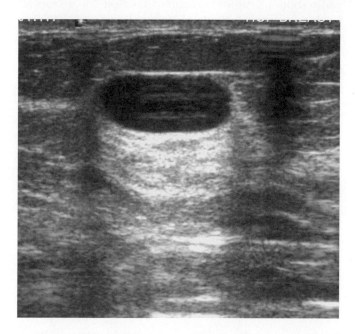

1. This 52-year-old woman presents with a palpable right breast mass. Describe the mammographic finding. If you had an ML view, would the mass move up or down in position relative to the position on the MLO? Where is the mass most likely located in the right breast?

2. Describe the ultrasound findings.

3. How accurate is ultrasound in the differentiation of a cyst vs a solid mass?

4. What are the echogenic horizontal lines in the anterior aspect of the lesion on ultrasound?

Cyst with Reverberation

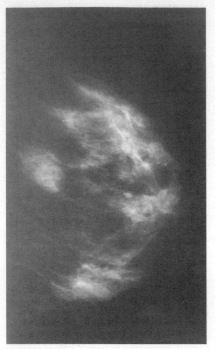

ML view

1. The high-density macrolobulated mass with partially obscured margins is located at approximately the 9 o'clock site in the right breast. Since the mass is slightly lateral on the CC view, it will move "down" on an ML or 90° lateral view relative to the MLO location.

2. Ultrasound shows a simple cyst with posterior acoustic enhancement and sharp margins.

3. When strict criteria are followed, ultrasound is almost 100% specific for differentiating simple cysts from solid masses.

4. An artifact—anterior reverberation.

Reference
Stavros TA: *Breast Ultrasound*, Philadelphia, 2004, Lippincott Williams & Wilkins.

Cross-Reference
Ikeda, *Breast Imaging: THE REQUISITES*, pp 41, 137.

Comment
The mass is partially obscured on the CC view but is in the lateral breast. On the MLO view, the mass projects slightly above the nipple axis. One could predict that on an ML or 90° lateral view, the mass would project slightly inferiorly relative to the position on the MLO view. Understanding this simple triangulation will help target

an ultrasound so that the mass may be further characterized.

Mammographically, this mass cannot be differentiated from a solid mass, such as a fibroadenoma, or a partially circumscribed solid mass, perhaps cancer. Ultrasound reveals that the mass is a simple cyst. When strict ultrasound criteria are used, the accuracy in differentiating simple cystic from solid masses is almost 100%. To meet the criteria of a simple cyst, the lesion must have smooth walls, sharp anterior and posterior borders, no internal echoes, and must demonstrate posterior acoustic enhancement. Occasionally, cysts are multiple or are clustered and may have thin internal septations. There should be no irregularity to the wall or mural nodules seen on thorough, careful scanning of the entire cyst.

This case demonstrates artifactual echoes in the anterior aspect of the cyst due to anterior reverberation from the gain being set too high. If "real" echoes are seen within a cyst, they may be due to benign debris or cholesterol crystals. These benign-type internal echoes are often seen to move when the cyst is agitated with manual compression. Solid mural nodules or thickened walls should prompt a recommendation for a biopsy. In this case, no further evaluation is needed because the cyst meets all the criteria for a simple cyst.

Notes

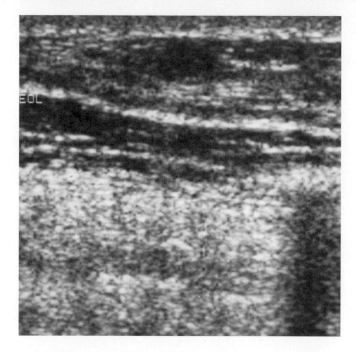 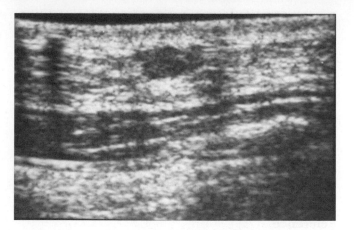

1. This 28-year-old woman presented with a breast lump in the periphery of the right breast. What is the first imaging study to be ordered?

2. Describe the ultrasound finding on the first image.

3. What change in instrumentation or imaging parameters may improve the evaluation of the superficial tissue?

4. Describe the findings on the second image.

Standoff Pad

1. Ultrasound, since the woman is younger than 30 years of age.

2. No definite abnormality is seen in the first ultrasound image of the superficial tissue.

3. The focal zone and depth should be corrected for near-field imaging. A standoff pad could also be used.

4. There is a slightly irregular subcentimeter mass. The finding is suspicious for malignancy.

Reference

Stavros TA: *Breast Ultrasound*, Philadelphia, 2004, Lippincott Williams & Wilkins.

Cross-Reference

Ikeda, *Breast Imaging: THE REQUISITES*, p 133.

Comment

The initial workup in this patient who is younger than 30 years of age should be a focused ultrasound examination of the area of palpable concern. The right axillary tail tissue was imaged, and since there is very little breast parenchyma in this area, the image on the left was obtained with a depth and focal zone focused deep near the muscle and ribs, but the image is not optimized for evaluation of the near field. The image on the right was obtained with the depth and the focal zones correctly placed in the superficial subcutaneous tissues of the very thin lateral breast. With this improved technique, a small irregular mass is evident. In a case such as this, because there is an irregular mass that is suspicious for malignancy seen on ultrasound, a mammogram should also be performed to assess for more extensive disease.

On ultrasound-guided core biopsy, this small irregular mass represented an invasive ductal carcinoma. If the ultrasound imaging had not been optimized with the correct placement of the focal zones, this small palpable mass would have been missed.

Notes

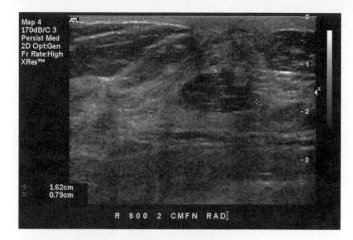

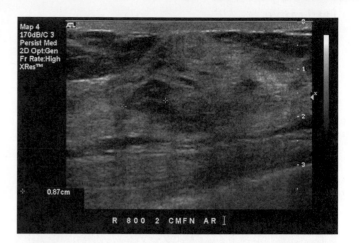

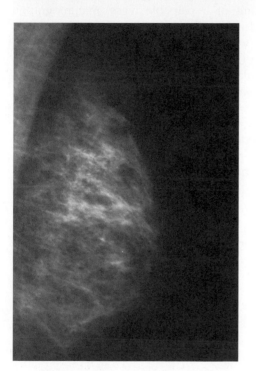

1. This is an ultrasound and mammogram of a 57-year-old who presented with a palpable finding in the subareolar right breast. Describe the ultrasound finding.

2. Does the ultrasound finding represent a suspicious mass?

3. Is there a mammographic abnormality in the subareolar right breast?

4. What are other ultrasound features of fat lobules to differentiate true masses?

Fat Lobule

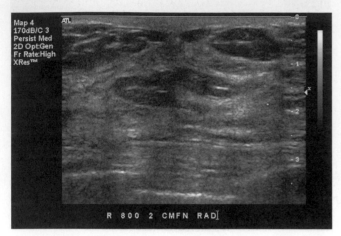

1. There is a hypoechoic area, isoechoic to fat in the subareolar right breast, surrounded by echogenic fibrous tissue.

2. This finding does not have suspicious criteria and is most compatible with a fat lobule. Look for a fat lobule to "spread out" in one plane, communicating with adjacent fat areas, rather than remaining as a mass on all planes.

3. No, the mammogram is normal.

4. The fat lobule contains thin, straight echogenic lines, parallel to the skin, which are fibrous septae that subdivide the lobule. The fat lobule should be compressible on increased pressure with the transducer.

References

Moy L, Slanetz PJ, Moore R, Satija S, Yeh ED, McCarthy KA, Hall D, Staffa M, Rafferty EA, Halpern E, Kopans DB: Specificity of mammography and US in the evaluation of a palpable abnormality: Retrospective review, *Radiology* 225(1):176–181, 2002.

Spencer GM, Rubens DJ, Roach DJ: Hypoechoic fat: A sonographic pitfall, *Am J Roentgenol* 164:1277–1280, 1995.

Venta LA, Dudiak CM, Salomon CG, Flisak ME: Sonographic evaluation of the breast, *RadioGraphics* 14:29–50, 1994.

Cross-Reference

Ikeda, *Breast Imaging: THE REQUISITES*, p 143.

Comment

The fat lobule seen on ultrasound can be confused with a solid mass, rendering a false-positive interpretation. Particularly in the setting of a palpable mass, you must be careful to be certain that what is being seen is fat and not a solid mass isoechoic to fat. Fat lobules can be palpable but should not be a firm suspicious mass.

When performing ultrasound, benign solid masses such as fibroadenoma can have an appearance similar to a fat lobule. Malignant masses usually have at least one characteristic, such as vertically oriented irregular margins, hyperechoic irregular rim, and shadowing. A fat lobule has none of these features. When a hypoechoic masslike structure is seen, orient the probe 90° to the original scan plane. If it is a fat lobule, it should merge with surrounding fat rather than have the appearance of a mass on both views. The fat lobule contains thin straight horizontal lines representing fibrous septae, not seen in malignant masses.

In the setting of a palpable mass, mammography should be performed. There are only a few exceptions to this rule: a woman who has had a mammogram in the recent past (<1 month) that is entirely normal, such as a fatty replaced breast, and a pregnant woman whose ultrasound is consistent with normal pregnancy-induced changes in the breast. (If the ultrasound is suspicious for cancer, mammogram should be done in the pregnant patient.) If the mammogram and ultrasound are normal, the predictive value that the area of concern is normal is almost 100%.

Notes

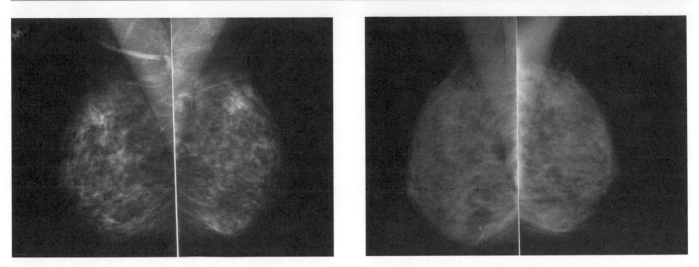

1. These two mammograms were taken 1 year apart, labeled with the same patient name. Is this the same person?

2. How can you explain the change in appearance of the breasts in the past year?

3. Why is it important to check the patient identity on the film?

4. How has weight loss contributed to the change in the mammographic appearance?

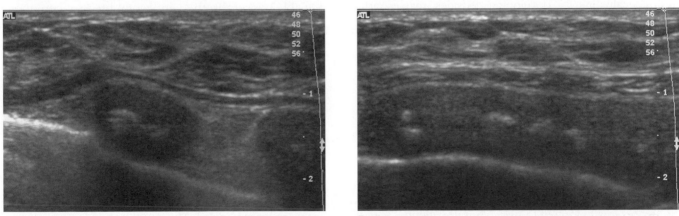

Antiradial   Radial

1. A 25-year-old patient presents with an area of palpable concern in her lateral breast. What initial study is chosen to workup the clinical findings?

2. Are there any suspicious findings on the ultrasound images provided?

3. What normal structure is seen in both the radial and the antiradial images that may be misconstrued as a mass?

4. What BI-RADS category is given for the ultrasound findings?

Weight Loss—Effect on Mammogram

1. These two mammograms are from the same patient.

2. The patient has had a significant weight loss.

3. Films can be mislabeled by the technologist. It is important to ensure that the mammograms are labeled correctly.

4. Weight loss results in the reduction of fat relative to gland tissue. The mammogram after weight loss has less fat, and the mammogram appears denser.

References

Stomper PC, D'Souza DJ, DiNitto PA: Analysis of parenchymal density on mammograms in 1353 women 25–79 years old, *Am J Roentgenol* 167:1261–1265, 1996.

Boyd NF, Greenberg C, Lockwood G, Little L, Martin L, Byng J, Yaffe M, Tritchler D: Effects at two years of a low-fat, high-carbohydrate diet on radiologic features of the breast: Results from a randomized trial. Canadian Diet and Breast Cancer Prevention Study Group, *J Natl Cancer Inst* 89(7):488–496, 1997.

Cross-Reference

Ikeda, *Breast Imaging: THE REQUISITES*, p 28.

Comment

It is important to assess interval change in the mammogram, comparing the current mammogram with previous exams, evaluating for developing densities, masses, and calcifications. In some instances, the entire exam may look very different than the previous mammogram. This may occur when the patient has begun or has stopped hormone replacement therapy or may occur in extreme weight loss, as in this case. This patient lost 63 pounds between the two mammograms (one-third of her initial weight). This caused a dramatic change in the appearance of the mammographic density. In the earlier exam, there are scattered glandular elements interspersed with fat. In the later exam, after the weight loss, the breasts appear much denser, and there is less contrast within the image. This change was dramatic enough to question whether the two exams belonged to two different patients.

When the appearance of the mammogram changes significantly, it underscores the importance of proper labeling of images. The patient's name and ID number are required to be indelibly located on each film (not on a label attached to the film). The technologist must check that the name is correct when viewing the final images, before letting the patient leave. When the films are hung for interpretation, the name is again checked. When the radiologist reads the mammogram, the name is checked again.

Notes

Ultrasound of Rib

1. An ultrasound is the first study to perform in a patient younger than 30 years of age.

2. No abnormality is seen in the breast parenchyma.

3. There are normal glandular structures as well as muscle and ribs seen. The rib may sometimes appear as a mass, but one must be careful to localize the rib below the pectoralis muscle.

4. This is a BI-RADS category 1: negative. Clinical correlation is recommended.

References

Dennis MA, Parker SH, Klaus AJ, Stavros AT, Kaske TI, Clark SB: Breast biopsy avoidance: The value of normal mammograms and normal sonograms in the setting of a palpable lump, *Radiology* 219:186–191, 2001.

Soo MS, Rosen EL, Baker JA, Vo TT, Boyd BA: Negative predictive value of sonography with mammography in patients with palpable breast lesions, *Am J Roentgenol* 177(5):1167–1170, 2001.

Cross-Reference

Ikeda, *Breast Imaging: THE REQUISITES*, p 136.

Comment

In this case, the young woman presents with an area of palpable concern in the very lateral breast where there is very little breast tissue. Imaging in the radial and anti-radial direction shows no abnormality in the breast parenchyma. There is visualization of the pectoralis muscle and the rib, and care must be taken to carefully image the breast parenchyma. The rib is a normal structure but may be misconstrued as a mass in the antiradial projection, where it is seen as "wider than tall" and demonstrates shadowing from the bone cortex. The location behind the pectoralis muscle and the longitudinal axis on the radial imaging proves that this is not a mass but rather the normal structure of the rib. Since no imaging finding is apparent, correlation with physical exam is recommended. The negative predictive value of ultrasound in this setting is almost 100%.

Notes

Fair Game

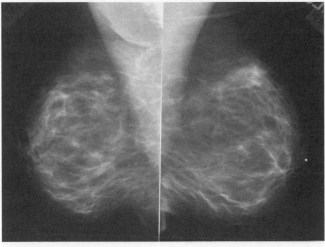

Initial

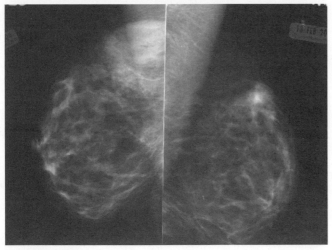

4 years later

1. What is the change between the two mammograms 4 years apart?

2. How would you proceed with the workup?

3. Is a biopsy needed?

4. Does MRI play a role?

Developing Asymmetric Glandular Tissue

1. A focal area of increased glandular density has developed in the left upper breast.

2. Spot compression views and ultrasound should be performed.

3. If no focal mass is identified on mammography or ultrasound, biopsy is not mandatory but may be desired for more complete evaluation.

4. MRI may be used instead of biopsy to evaluate for abnormal enhancement in this area.

References

Homer MJ, Smith TJ: Asymmetric breast tissue, *Radiology* 173:577–578, 1989.

Piccoli CW, Feig SA, Palazzo JP: Developing asymmetric breast tissue, *Radiology* 211(1):111–117, 1999.

Samardar P, de Paredes ES, Grimes MM, Wilson JD: Focal asymmetric densities seen at mammography: US and pathologic correlation, *RadioGraphics* 22(1):19–33, 2002.

Cross-Reference

Ikeda, *Breast Imaging: THE REQUISITES*, p 30.

Comment

Focal asymmetry is described in the BI-RADS lexicon as "visible as asymmetry of tissue density with similar shape on two views, but completely lacking borders and the conspicuity of a true mass." Focal asymmetry is not unusual on the routine mammogram; it is reportedly seen in 3% of women. Although it can be normal, developing asymmetric areas can also be a sign of malignancy and so must be viewed with caution and evaluated thoroughly.

It is important to review all the previous mammograms. If the previous mammograms are at a different site, there is value in obtaining them. If the area is stable compared to prior films, no further workup is needed.

In this patient, the asymmetry is new. Features of malignancy must be sought: Are the borders convex? Are the borders spiculated? Are there calcifications? Additional views can be done to determine if the tissue spreads out, and you can look through the tissue for interspersed fat, a benign feature. The additional views could include spot compression and rolled craniocaudal view and/or a true lateral view. Ultrasound is a very good tool for evaluating focal asymmetry. The classic ultrasound appearance is that of hyperechoic dense fibrous tissue with ducts coursing through. There should be no mass, distortion, or abnormal area of shadowing.

A core biopsy can be performed if there is concern by the patient, or if the asymmetry is palpable. The histology is often stromal fibrosis or pseudoangiomatous stromal hyperplasia. MRI can be done instead of needle biopsy. On MRI, the enhancement of the asymmetric tissue should be the same as that of the rest of the gland tissue in the breast, with no abnormal enhancement.

Notes

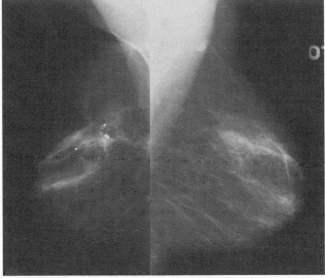

MLOs

CCs

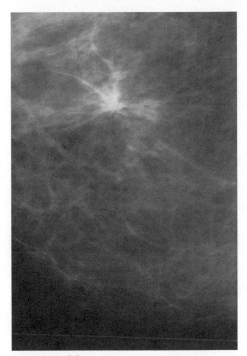

Spot of left CC

1. This patient has had a left lumpectomy (in the upper outer quadrant), left axillary dissection, and radiation therapy. Describe the finding in the left medial breast best seen on the CC view (see spot magnification view).

2. What is the most likely diagnosis? What history should you ask the patient?

3. What BI-RADS category should this be?

4. What is the final assessment category?

Scar—Importance of Old Films

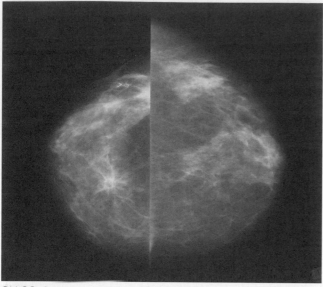

Old CC views

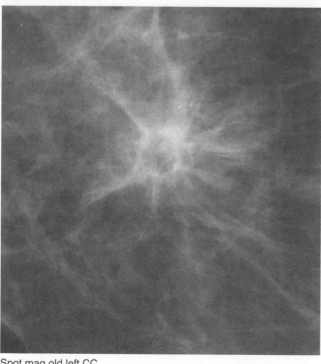

Spot mag old left CC

1. There is a small spiculated mass in the medial left breast.

2. This could represent a new malignancy, but the patient should be questioned to determine if there has been any surgery in this area or if there are old films for comparison.

3. If there are old films that may be obtained but are not available at the time of her diagnostic mammogram, the case should be BI-RADS category 0.

4. "Incomplete, comparison with prior films needed."

Cross-Reference
Ikeda, *Breast Imaging: THE REQUISITES*, pp 39, 110.

Comment
This case demonstrates the importance of obtaining all pertinent history from the patient at the time of the study and the importance of obtaining old films. This patient did not remember that she had had a biopsy in the medial left breast, and there was no visible skin scar for the technologist to make note of or question the patient about. The patient does have significant distortion in the site of her prior lumpectomy in the upper outer quadrant of the left breast. If the patient has had prior films, they should be obtained prior to making a final decision about the finding in the medial breast. This patient's films were at another institution, and the case had to remain a category 0: incomplete, until the prior films were obtained and compared.

When the prior films were obtained, it was immediately evident that the spiculated area in the medial left breast was due to a prior surgical biopsy. The earlier images (left) show an area of architectural distortion with a central lucency consistent with fat necrosis. The change over time is that of further healing and retraction of the scar tissue. Although the current images are concerning for a small spiculated cancer in the medial left breast, the comparison with the older films demonstrated that the area of distortion is actually smaller and resolving, consistent with a benign change. Having the older films for comparison in this case was essential, and a biopsy was avoided. After comparison with the prior films, the case was addended and changed to a BI-RADS category 2: benign. Routine follow-up was recommended.

Notes

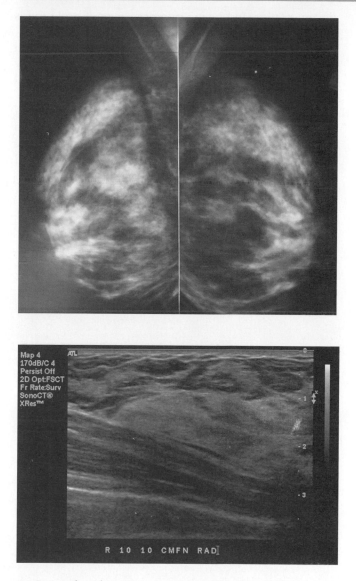

1. Describe the mammogram for this young woman with a palpable lump in the right upper outer breast.

2. What is the next imaging step?

3. If the mammogram and ultrasound are normal, what is the next step?

4. Does the referring physician need to be informed immediately of your findings?

Predictive Value of Negative Mammogram and Ultrasound

1. The glandular tissue is heterogeneously dense. No abnormality is seen.

2. Ultrasound and a clinical exam directed to the palpable finding should be performed.

3. Report the imaging findings as negative, and then you may recommend clinical follow-up based on clinical exam by the referring physician. Decision to biopsy may be made on clinical grounds alone.

4. It is important to communicate the results of a palpable concern to the referring physician on the same day as the workup if the results are suspicious.

References

Dennis MA: Breast biopsy avoidance: The value of normal mammograms and normal sonograms in the setting of palpable lump, *Radiology* 219:186–191, 2001.

Moy L, Slanetz PJ, Moore R, Satija S, Yeh ED, McCarthy KA, Hall D, Staffa M, Rafferty EA, Halpern E, Kopans DB: Specificity of mammography and US in the evaluation of a palpable abnormality, *Retrospective Rev Radiol* 225:176–181, 2002.

Shetty MK, et al.: Prospective evaluation of the value of combined mammographic and sonographic assessment in patients with palpable abnormalities of the breast, *J Ultrasound Med* 22:263–268, 2003.

Cross-Reference

Ikeda, *Breast Imaging: THE REQUISITES*, p 150.

Comment

This patient presents with a palpable finding on her referring physician's exam in the left upper outer breast. This is her baseline mammogram at age 38. No abnormality is seen.

An ultrasound is the next imaging study to be performed. At the time of the ultrasound, examine the area clinically. Ask the patient to show you the area of concern. Sometimes, the patient cannot give you an exact area, particularly if the referring physician noted the abnormality, not the patient. Then perform ultrasound, looking for a cyst, a mass, or an area of distortion.

There may be no evidence of a focal finding to explain the palpable area. What you may find is a region of hyperechoic gland tissue surrounded by hypoechoic fat. This may feel prominent on the clinical exam. This is quite commonly the case, and it is a reliable negative finding. Images should be obtained of the area for documentation and billing purposes, even if no lesion is identified with ultrasound.

The predictive value of negative mammogram and negative ultrasound exams in the setting of a clinically palpable finding was found to be nearly 100% in several studies.

The report should delineate the results of the imaging performed, and you may advise the referring physician of the reliability of the negative imaging findings. The referring physician may choose to recommend biopsy of the palpable finding based on clinical grounds alone.

Notes

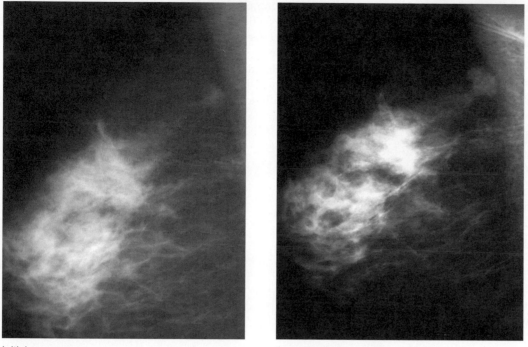

Initial mammogram   1 year later

1. Is there a suspicious finding on the initial left MLO view?

2. Is there a suspicious finding on the left MLO view one year later?

3. What are the reasons that the mass was overlooked initially?

4. How can false-negative mammograms be reduced?

False Negative—Missed Cancer

1. There is a suspicious spiculated 1-cm mass in the upper outer quadrant on the left MLO view, posteriorly, in the upper breast.

2. The suspicious mass has markedly increased in size since the previous exam, consistent with malignancy.

3. The mass on the initial exam is in the axillary tail of the breast, at the edge of the film, and is seen only on one view. Anteriorly, there is dense breast tissue, which may have distracted the reader.

4. False-negative exams can be reduced by education in what early cancer looks like, by training the radiologist to use a systematic approach, by checking target areas more likely to harbor cancer in the upper outer quadrant, and by checking the edge of the glandular tissue. Double reading of the mammogram, by using a second radiologist or by using computer-aided detection, has also been shown to reduce the false-negative mammogram.

References

Ikeda DM, Birdwell RL, O'Shaughnessy KF, Brenner RJ, Sickles EA: Analysis of 172 subtle findings on prior normal mammograms in women with breast cancer detected at follow-up screening, *Radiology* 226: 494–503, 2003.

Thurfjell EL, Lernevall KA, Taube AA: Benefit of independent double reading in a population-based mammography screening program, *Radiology* 191:241, 1994.

Cross-Reference

Ikeda, *Breast Imaging: THE REQUISITES*, pp 315–316.

Comment

The false-negative mammogram is a significant problem. It is very difficult or impossible to detect all early cancers, but an effort must be made to reduce the miss rate of potentially detectable lesions. Education about the varied mammographic appearance of early cancers and where they are more likely to be located can help. Improving the technical quality of the mammogram is important because a suboptimal technique will limit the exam. The dense breast can be distracting, particularly if other lesions are present. A small mass may be overlooked because of its size. A lesion in the axilla may be mistaken for a normal lymph node.

The environment in which the radiologist interprets exams is important. Screening mammograms (these two exams were both screening exams; no mass was felt) should be read in a controlled environment, with little outside interruptions, and by radiologists who read mammograms routinely. Double reading or computer-aided detection of screening mammograms has been shown to decrease the miss rate of early cancers 7–15% and, if time and staffing allow, may be a viable option.

Despite all efforts to detect cancer in the breast, cancers will be missed. Reviewing the missed cancers can help train the radiologist in improved detection.

Notes

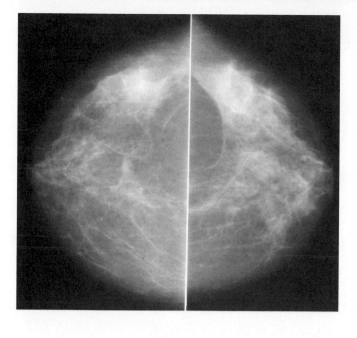

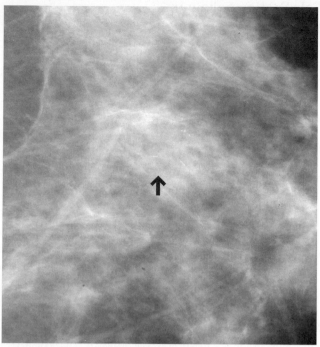

Right mag CC

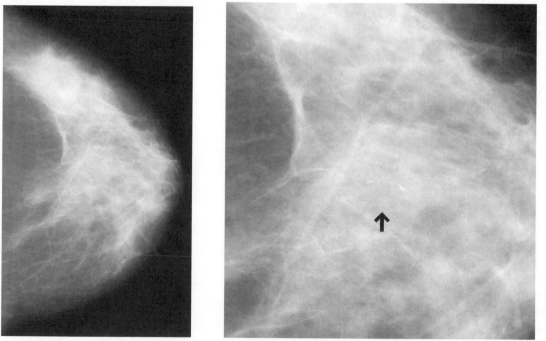

6 months later

Mag CC 6 months later

1. A 47-year-old presents for a screening mammography and is recalled for additional imaging of a small cluster of right breast calcifications, best seen on the CC view (*arrows*). What is the BI-RADS category at screening? What is the overall impression?

2. On recall, a few calcifications are seen on magnification views and a short-term follow-up is recommended. What BI-RADS category is given? What overall assessment is given?

3. What should the likelihood of malignancy be for a BI-RADS category 3 case?

4. How long should the patient be followed at short intervals?

Calcification Follow-up

1. BI-RADS category 0: incomplete, additional imaging is needed. The overall assessment: Incomplete.

2. Category 3: probably benign, short-term follow-up is recommended. The overall assessment: Probably benign.

3. The interpreting radiologist should believe that there is a very low likelihood of malignancy—less than 2%.

4. The patient should be followed closely at 6-month intervals and since faint calcifications are the concern, magnification views should be performed at follow-up. Close follow-up for calcifications thought to be "probably benign" is generally performed at 6-month intervals for 2 years unless there is a change that is concerning, in which case a biopsy is recommended.

References

Orel SG, Kay N, Reynolds C, Sullivan DC: BI-RADS categorization as a predictor of malignancy, *Radiology* 211:845, 1999.

Rosen EL, Baker JA, Scott Soo M: Malignant lesions initially subjected to short-term mammographic follow-up, *Radiology* 223:221, 2002.

Vizcaino I, Gadea L, Andreo L, Salas D, Ruiz-Perales F, Cuevas D, Herranz C, Bueno F: Short-term follow-up results in 795 nonpalpable probably benign lesions detected at screening mammography, *Radiology* 219:475, 2001.

Cross-Reference

Ikeda, *Breast Imaging: THE REQUISITES*, p 84.

Comment

When the screening study was interpreted and the patient was to be called back, the appropriate BI-RADS category is 0: incomplete. After the patient is called back for the magnification views and the calcifications are thought to be most likely due to a benign process, the BI-RADS is category 3: probably benign, short-term follow-up recommended. A 6-month follow-up with magnification views is recommended of the right breast only. However, at 6 months when the patient returned for follow-up, the calcifications had changed significantly and a biopsy was recommended. Biopsy revealed that the calcifications were due to a high-grade comedo DCIS.

In assessing calcifications, magnification views are very important because background faint calcifications may be evident that are not seen on routine imaging. There is no magic number of calcifications for which a biopsy is needed. More important are the morphology and distribution of the calcifications and if they are new. In this case, on the baseline study the calcifications were thought to be punctate and due to a probably benign process rather than linear or pleomorphic, which are more concerning morphologies. However, in 6 months, the calcifications changed significantly. They had increased in number, and linear forms were evident. Stereotactic core biopsy was performed and DCIS was found. The patient then went on to definitive lumpectomy and radiation therapy.

A short-term follow-up should only be used when a lesion is thought to be most likely benign. One series suggests that if a lesion is placed in category 3: probably benign, the likelihood of malignancy in the reader's mind for the lesion should be very low, less than 2%. Others suggest that the threshold for short-term follow-up should be even lower, less than 1%, since percutaneous biopsies are easy to do and relatively risk free.

Notes

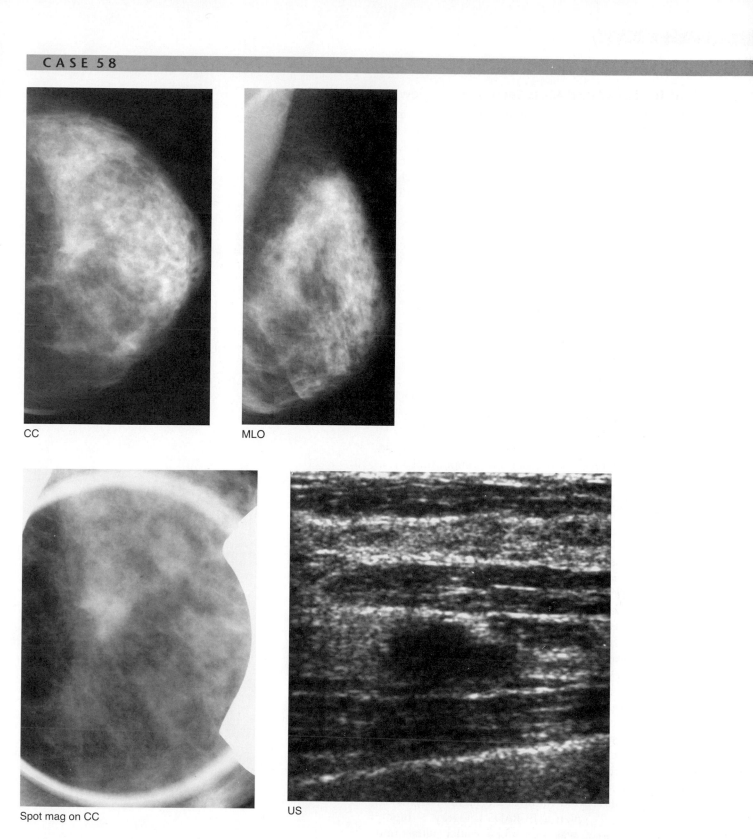

CC

MLO

Spot mag on CC

US

1. A dense focal asymmetry is seen on the cranial caudad view in the posterior central aspect of the right breast. No definite abnormality is seen on the MLO view. What is the next imaging step?

2. The focal asymmetry appears irregular on the spot view but no abnormality is seen on the lateral view. What is the next imaging step?

3. At what location in the breast would one look for this lesion with ultrasound?

4. What BI-RADS category would be given based on the combined mammographic and ultrasound findings?

Hunt for Spiculated Mass Seen on One View

1. A spot magnification view in the CC projection is needed to assess if the focal asymmetry is "real" or just due to a superimposition of normal tissue. The spot view may also help evaluate the margins of any possible mass. A straight lateral view may also be helpful to triangulate the location of a possible lesion.

2. Ultrasound is recommended.

3. Since the area is seen centrally on the cranial caudad view, targeted ultrasound evaluation should be performed at the 6 and 12 o'clock sites.

4. Ultrasound reveals a hypoechoic irregular mass deep against the pectoralis muscle. BI-RADS category 5: highly suspicious, biopsy necessary.

Cross-Reference
Ikeda, *Breast Imaging: THE REQUISITES*, pp 46, 92.

Comment
The finding of an abnormality seen on only a single mammographic projection is not uncommon. Initially, a spot compression view is obtained to determine if a lesion actually persists with compression and to analyze the margins if a persistent abnormality is seen. In this case, the spot compression brought out the spiculation associated with this mass and made the appearance even more suspicious. (The desmoplastic reaction of the cancer is accentuated on spot compression views.) The next step in the imaging workup would be to triangulate the exact location of the suspicious mass so that a directed ultrasound, and eventually biopsy, is possible. A straight lateral view was obtained but no discreet abnormality was seen. Rolled views in the cranial caudad projection might also be helpful in some cases.

For further evaluation and to localize the lesion, an ultrasound would be the next step. Since the spiculated mass is seen deep and central on the cranial caudad view, the ultrasound should be directed at the 6 and 12 o'clock sites, deep near the chest wall. On ultrasound, an irregular, hypoechoic mass abutting the pectoralis muscle is seen. The combined mammographic and ultrasound findings are highly suspicious, and this lesion is given a BI-RADS category 5: highly suspicious. Biopsy was performed under ultrasound guidance and this proved to be an invasive ductal carcinoma.

Notes

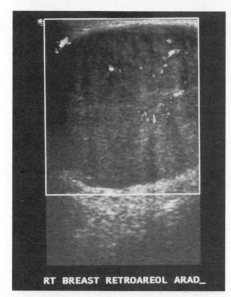

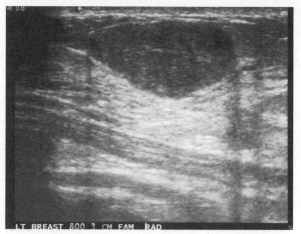

RT BREAST RETROAREOL ARAD_

Dominant mass

LT BREAST 800 3 CM FAM RAD

Smaller additional mass

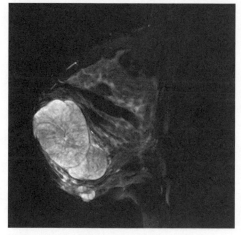

Fat suppressed T2 images

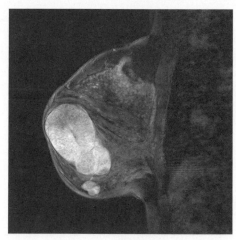

Post GD

1. Describe the ultrasound and MRI findings in this 16-year-old with asymmetric breast enlargement.
2. Is a mammographic workup necessary?
3. What is the differential diagnosis and appropriate management of this lesion?
4. Are there management issues regarding the contralateral breast?

Juvenile Fibroadenoma

1. The ultrasound shows a very large, well-circumscribed, mixed echotecture solid mass. The mass has a high signal on T2 and is highly vascular on MRI. Other smaller solid masses are seen in the surrounding tissue.

2. Mammography is not necessary in this 16-year-old. The lesion is well demonstrated on ultrasound and there is no need for screening the rest of the breast for cancer since the incidence is extremely low in this age group.

3. The lesion is most likely a giant or juvenile fibroadenoma. Because of the significant asymmetry of the breast, surgical excision is recommended for cosmetic reasons.

4. An MRI is recommended of both breasts to establish a baseline of size and location of possible additional lesions.

References

Orel SG, Schnall MD: MR imaging of the breast for the detection, diagnosis, and staging of breast cancer, *Radiology* 220:13–30, 2001.

Weinstein SP, Conant EF, Orel SG, Zuckerman JA, Bellah R: Spectrum of US findings in pediatric and adolescent patients with palpable breast masses, *RadioGraphics* 20:1613–1621, 2000.

White Nunes L, Schnall MD, Orel SG, Hochman MG, Langlotz CP, Reynolds CA, Torosian MH: Correlation of lesion appearance and histologic findings for the nodes of a breast MR imaging interpretation model, *RadioGraphics* 19:79–92, 1999.

Cross-Reference

Ikeda, *Breast Imaging: THE REQUISITES*, pp 110, 205.

Comment

The workup was initiated with an ultrasound because of the patient's young age. A mammogram is unnecessary since the likelihood of cancer is extremely low and the lesion appears so benign. On ultrasound, there is a well-circumscribed large mass that has small internal cystic areas. On the T2 fat-suppressed MRI, the large mass has a very high signal and shows steady, progressive enhancement. Fibrovascular septa are visible as black bands coursing through the mass. The most common solid mass in this age group is a fibroadenoma. In young girls or teens, rapidly growing fibroadenomas may be called juvenile or giant fibroadenomas. In this teenager with a very large fibroadenoma, surgical excision was desired for cosmetic reasons. If the surgical excision is not performed, biopsy of such a large dominant mass is necessary to exclude the rare phyllodes tumor, which is locally aggressive and occasionally may metastasize.

Fibroadenomas are multiple in approximately 20% of patients. A bilateral ultrasound or MRI is helpful in this patient to map out and provide a baseline image of any other lesion in the breast of concern as well as the contralateral breast. Not all these classically benign smaller masses need to be biopsied, but establishing a baseline imaging study is helpful to allow clinical follow-up. No further imaging follow-up is needed of the other masses, but if the young woman presents with additional masses in the future, the MRI may be used to establish if there is interval growth. Occasionally, masses that have been stable on imaging present as "newly palpable" because a new health care provider is doing a breast exam.

Notes

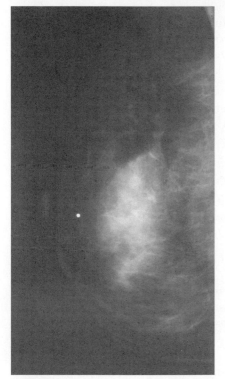

MLO view

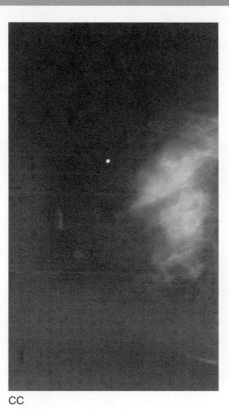

CC

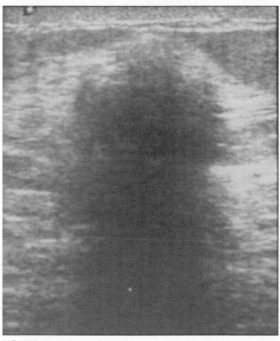

US rad

1. This 40-year-old juvenile-onset diabetic has a new palpable mass. Describe the mammographic and ultrasound findings.

2. What is the appropriate BI-RADS category and assessment? What is the differential diagnosis?

3. What type of biopsy is recommended?

4. What other systemic complications are often seen in these patients?

CASE 60

Diabetic Mastopathy

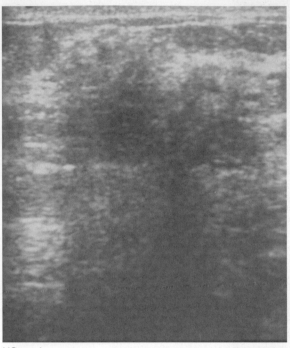

US arad

1. There is a focal asymmetry in the left breast. This is not a mammographic mass because it does not have convex margins on two views. Ultrasound, however, does reveal an irregular solid mass associated with shadowing.

2. Category 4, suspicious. Biopsy is recommended to exclude malignancy. The differential diagnosis includes diabetic mastopathy and invasive breast carcinoma.

3. The diagnosis of diabetic mastopathy was made by ultrasound-guided core biopsy.

4. Patients with diabetic mastopathy generally have long-standing juvenile-onset diabetes and have the associated complications of that disease.

Reference

Weinstein SP, Conant EF, Orel SG, Lawton TJ, Acs G: Diabetic mastopathy in men: Imaging findings in two patients, *Radiology* 219:797, 2001.

Cross-Reference

Ikeda, *Breast Imaging: THE REQUISITES,* pp 308–309.

Comment

Diabetic mastopathy is an uncommon condition occurring in patients with long-standing insulin-dependent diabetes. It is most often diagnosed in premenopausal women but has been reported in men. The most common presentation is a new firm palpable mass that may mimic carcinoma on breast exam. Patients frequently have associated complications from their diabetes, such as renal disease, retinopathy, and cardiac disease.

The mammographic findings in diabetic mastopathy are usually a poorly defined mass or a dense focal asymmetry; patients frequently have mammographically detected vascular calcifications as a complication of their long-standing diabetes. However, since many of these patients are young, the mass may not be mammographically visible due to surrounding dense breast tissue. Ultrasound may demonstrate a poorly defined mass or just areas of intense acoustic shadowing.

With the appropriate clinical history and the sonographic features, the diagnosis of diabetic mastopathy may be suggested, but tissue diagnosis is necessary to exclude malignancy. Core biopsy reveals thick bundles of collagen and periductal, lobular, and vascular inflammatory infiltrates. An autoimmune etiology has been postulated for this condition.

Notes

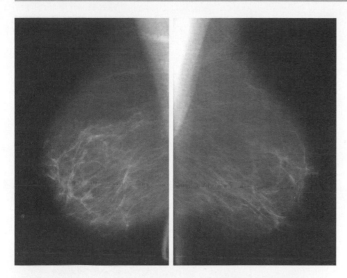
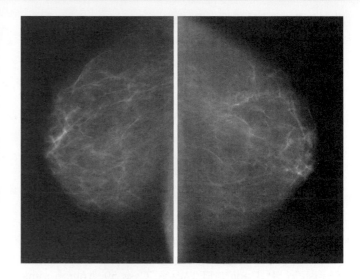

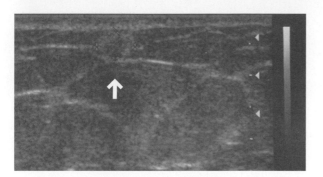

1. This patient presents with a palpable mass in the left upper inner breast. What additional imaging studies are needed?

2. Is there any additional history that is important?

3. What is in your differential diagnosis?

4. Are the ultrasound features suspicious for malignancy?

Angiolipoma of the Breast

1. Spot compression views, tangential views with BB marker and ultrasound.

2. Yes—any history of trauma or bruising.

3. Hematoma, lipoma, hemangioma, angiolipoma, and angiosarcoma.

4. The ultrasound features are not typically benign. Biopsy is indicated because of the sonographic appearance and because it is palpable.

References

Stavros AT, et al.: Solid breast nodules: Use of sonography to distinguish between benign and malignant lesions, *Radiology* 196:123–134, 1995.

Weinstein SP, Conant EF, Acs G: Case 59: Angiolipoma of the breast, *Radiology* 227:773–775, 2003.

Cross-Reference

Ikeda, *Breast Imaging: THE REQUISITES*, p 134.

Comment

This patient presents with a palpable, superficial mass. On the mammogram, there is a low-density mass with circumscribed margins. It persists on spot compression views. Ultrasound shows a mass directly beneath the skin. The margins of the mass are microlobulated, and there is a thick irregular hyperechoic capsule. These features are suspicious for malignancy. The skin surface is normal.

The patient related no history of trauma. However, a common presentation after trauma is a palpable mass, a hematoma, that may have an identical appearance on mammography and ultrasound. Careful questioning of the patient for any history of recent trauma is helpful, as is examination of the breast for signs of bruising. If the clinical presentation is consistent with trauma, no biopsy is necessary. The patient can be asked to return for follow-up in 6–8 weeks, and if the mass resolves completely, no further evaluation is needed. Trauma can cause an occult breast malignancy to present as a palpable concern if the mass bleeds and enlarges.

This patient underwent a needle core biopsy using vacuum technique, and the histology report was that of an unusual vascular lesion, with cellular atypia and mitotic activity, most consistent with cellular angiolipoma. Excision of the remainder of the mass was advised to exclude angiosarcoma. The histology of the excised specimen was cellular angiolipoma of the subcutis, and no malignant transformation was seen. This is an unusual tumor of the breast, more typically seen in the back, neck, and shoulder.

Notes

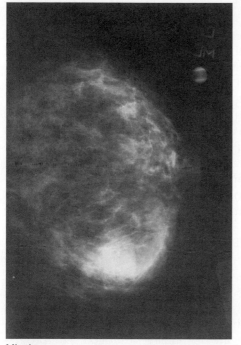

ML view

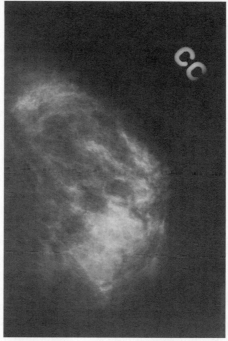

CC view

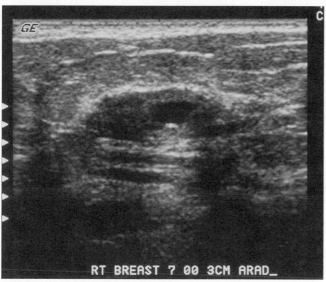

US

1. This 45-year-old woman presented with a new palpable lump. What are the necessary imaging steps?

2. Describe the ultrasound and mammographic findings and give a BI-RADS category.

3. What is the most likely diagnosis?

4. Core biopsy yields pseudoangiogiomatous stromal hyperplasia (PASH). What is the appropriate management?

PASH

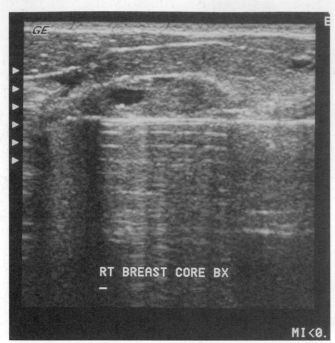

RT BREAST CORE BX

1. A mammogram should be performed initially, preferably with a BB on the area of palpable concern (this was not done in this case). Targeted ultrasound is also needed to evaluate the area of palpable concern.

2. Ultrasound demonstrates a solid well-defined, macrolobulated, hypoechoic mass that has internal cystic spaces. BI-RADS category 4: biopsy is recommended.

3. Fibroadenoma, or other benign fibroepithelial lesion and phyllodes tumor.

4. PASH is a benign stromal proliferation.

References

Cohen MA, Morris EA, Rosen PP, Dershaw DD, Liberman L, Abramson AF: Pseudoangiomatous stromal hyperplasia: Mammographic, sonographic, and clinical patterns, *Radiology* 198:117, 1996.

Stavros AT, et al.: Solid breast nodules: Use of sonography to distinguish between benign and malignant lesions, *Radiology* 196:123–134, 1995.

Cross-Reference

Ikeda, *Breast Imaging: THE REQUISITES*, p 118.

Comment

The mammogram in this case reveals a focal asymmetry in the medial breast that corresponds in location and size with the area of palpable concern. The mammographic appearance is nonspecific. There is no distortion or suspicious calcifications, but ultrasound is needed for further characterization of the area of concern. Ultrasound demonstrates a well-defined mass that has internal cystic spaces and is macrolobulated. According to the Stavros criteria for characterizing solid mass with ultrasound, this is most likely a benign mass, probably a fibroadenoma. A biopsy was performed because the mass was large and according to the patient had grown over time. Biopsy revealed the benign histologic condition, pseudoangiomatous stromal hyperplasia (PASH).

PASH was first described in 1986 as a clinicopathologic entity consisting of a localized stromal proliferation that may form a discrete, painless, often palpable breast mass in premenopausal women. The most frequent clinical diagnosis is fibroadenoma, and on imaging, the appearance may be very similar. The etiology of PASH is unknown, although it is usually seen in premenopausal women as a mass-forming process and, more commonly, as a focal stromal change on biopsy. Studies have shown that PASH is hormonally responsive and there are identifiable estrogen and progesterone receptors. The diagnosis of PASH may be made on core biopsy, as in this case. No further evaluation is necessary, and after confirmation of the benign histology, the patient was returned to routine follow-up.

Notes

1. A 15-year-old give presents with a solitary breast mass. What is the best method of imaging to use?

2. Is this mass cystic or solid?

3. How would you manage a palpable cyst?

4. What is the management for this lesion?

Breast Mass in Teenager

1. Ultrasound is the best method of imaging in this age group. Mammography is not indicated.

2. This mass is solid.

3. No further evaluation is necessary for a simple cyst; however, a palpable cyst can be aspirated if the patient elects.

4. There are options in the management of this solid mass. Since it has benign features, the patient may elect to follow. Needle core biopsy could be performed for histologic diagnosis. Surgical excision is a reasonable choice since the mass may continue to grow.

References

Kronemer KA: Gray scale sonography of breast masses in adolescent girls, *J Ultrasound Med* 20(8):881, 2001.

Stavros AT, et al.: Solid breast nodules: Use of sonography to distinguish between benign and malignant, *Radiology* 196(1):123, 1995.

Cross-Reference

Ikeda, *Breast Imaging: THE REQUISITES*, p 150.

Comment

Ultrasound is the imaging method of choice in the young since it uses no ionizing radiation. When evaluating the patient with a lump, have the patient point to the area of concern. Ultrasound is used to determine if the palpable finding is cystic or solid. A solid mass may be hypoechoic or isoechoic to neighboring fat. When evaluating a solid mass, look for features that help characterize the lesion as benign or malignant. These characteristics include margin analysis, acoustic shadowing, and echotexture. Benign masses are oval, gently lobulated, parallel to the skin, and sharply circumscribed.

In this patient, there is an hypoechoic mass with gentle lobulations and sharply circumscribed borders, corresponding to the palpable finding. It is most consistent with a fibroadenoma.

The fibroadenoma is a common benign mass of the breast, occurring in 10–25% of women. The mass arises from the breast lobule and is most likely stimulated by estrogen. Fibroadenomas occur as multiple masses in approximately 20% of cases. Histologically, there is a fibrous stroma without cytologic atypia, and there is also an epithelial component. Morphologically, they are circumscribed round, oval, or bilobed, and they can occur anywhere in the breast.

In a study of 57 masses in adolescent girls (median age, 15.4 years), 36 masses were fibroadenoma. All masses were benign. Malignancy is extremely rare in this age group.

Because malignancy is unusual, there are options in the management of the solid mass in the adolescent breast. Traditionally, excisional biopsy was performed. It is now acceptable to follow the mass, once benign characteristics have been established with ultrasound evaluation. If there is growth, excision is recommended. If knowledge of the histology is desired but surgery is not, needle core biopsy gives a reliable histological diagnosis. In this patient, excision was performed and the mass was a fibroadenoma.

Notes

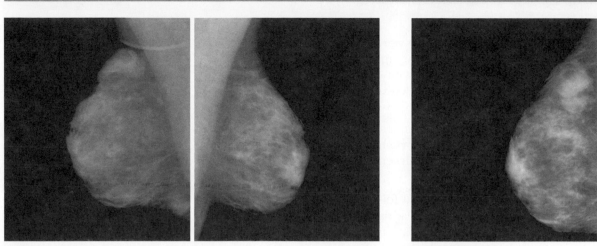

MLOs   Rotated lateral CC

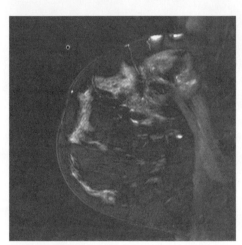   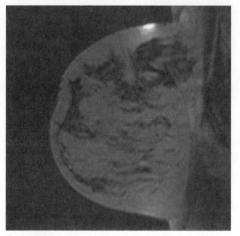

Post contrast   T1 image

1. This patient presented with an area of palpable thickening in the upper outer quadrant of her left breast. Describe the mammographic findings.

2. What additional imaging might be helpful?

3. Ultrasound imaging was negative and an MRI was recommended. Describe the finding on MRI. What is this most likely due to?

4. What BI-RADS category should be given?

Focal Asymmetry

1. A rotated cranial caudad view and the MLO view of the left breast show a focal asymmetry in the upper outer quadrant of the breast. The area of asymmetry has a mixed density and there is no evidence of architectural distortion.

2. An ultrasound would be the next step to make sure that there is not a mass or any suspicious imaging finding that corresponds with the area of thickening.

3. The MRI shows an enhancement pattern that follows enhancement of the remaining glandular tissue. No suspicious findings are seen by MRI. This focal asymmetry most likely represents an island of normal asymmetric breast tissue.

4. A BI-RADS category 2: benign, no evidence of malignancy.

References

Piccoli CW, Feig SA, Palazzo JP: Developing asymmetric breast tissue, *Radiology* 211(1):111–117, 1999.

Samardar P, Shaw de Paredes E, Grimes MM, Wilson JD: Focal asymmetric densities seen at mammography: US and pathologic correlation, *RadioGraphics* 22:19, 2002.

Cross-Reference

Ikeda, *Breast Imaging: THE REQUISITES*, p 37.

Comment

This patient presented with an area of palpable concern. Multiple mammographic views were performed, and the focal asymmetry in the upper outer quadrant of the left breast had an appearance most consistent with glandular tissue. However, since this area was palpable, an ultrasound was performed. No suspicious solid mass or area of architectural distortion was evident on ultrasound but, rather, normal glandular and ductal structures were seen. Because this area was of palpable concern to the patient, an MRI was recommended for further evaluation. The MRI showed a normal pattern of glandular enhancement in the area of the focal asymmetry. No suspicious findings were seen on MRI. The combination of the normal ultrasound, the mixed density area on mammography, and the normal MRI findings suggests that this is an island of asymmetric glandular tissue. Although close follow-up is recommended with physical exam, no further imaging evaluation is needed and a biopsy is unnecessary.

Notes

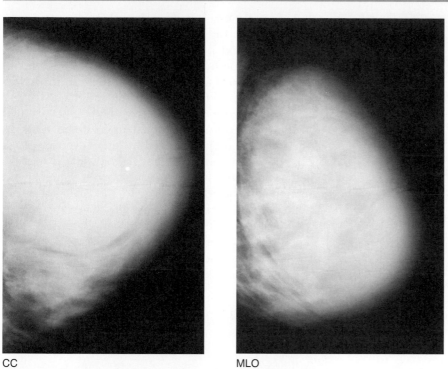

CC   MLO

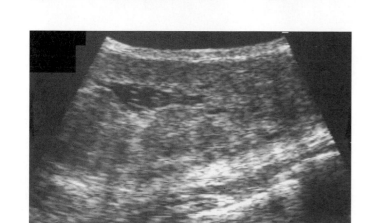

US

1. This 38-year-old patient is recently postpartum and presents with a very large palpable mass in the right breast. The mass began growing rapidly in her second trimester of pregnancy and measures approximately 12 cm on exam. How should the imaging workup begin?

2. Describe the mammographic and ultrasound findings.

3. What is the differential diagnosis for this mass?

4. What is the natural history of these benign masses?

Lactating Adenoma

1. A mammogram followed by an ultrasound.

2. Mammographically, the breast is extremely dense and the mass is almost completely obscured by the dense breast tissue. However, there is a suggestion of a sharp margin of the mass medially on the CC view. The ultrasound image shows only a portion of the mass, but it is solid, has a heterogeneous texture, and has large internal cystic areas.

3. This most likely represents a benign lactating adenoma or fibroadenoma.

4. A biopsy was requested by the patient and the referring physician because of the large size and rapid growth. The imaging appearance and clinical history are very consistent with a benign lactating adenoma and the mass could be followed. After pregnancy and cessation of nursing, these lesions frequently resolve or significantly decrease in size and excision is unnecessary.

References

Cardenosa G: *The Core Curriculum: Breast Imaging,* Philadelphia, 2004, Lippincott Williams & Wilkins, p 221.

Sumkin JH, Perrone AM, Harris KM, Nath ME, Amortegui AJ, Weinstein BJ: Lactating adenoma: US features and literature review, *Radiology* 206:271, 1998.

Cross-Reference

Ikeda, *Breast Imaging: THE REQUISITES*, p 116.

Comment

The main differential diagnosis for a palpable solid breast mass in the pregnant or lactating female is fibroadenoma, lactational adenoma, tubular adenoma, focal mastitis, galactocele, normal breast tissue with lactational changes (lobular hyperplasia), and of course, cancer is possible.

This patient had a lactational adenoma. These benign stromal tumors typically present during pregnancy as palpable mobile masses that undergo rapid growth. Often, a mammogram is not necessary because of the young age of the patient (<30 years) or because the patient presents during pregnancy.

Mammographically, the masses may be quite large. If the patient is lactating, the breast may be so dense that the masses cannot be well differentiated from the surrounding glandular tissue. On ultrasound, these masses are frequently well-defined hypoechoic solid masses with macrolobulation and have the long axis parallel to the chest wall. Frequently, ultrasound may also show large cystic areas, as in this case. Because of the uniform internal contents, there is often posterior acoustic enhancement. Occasionally, lactational adenomas may have indistinct or irregular margins, heterogeneous echotextures, and posterior acoustic shadowing, making the distinction from a malignant mass more difficult. This rapidly growing but benign-appearing mass was highly vascular, and because of the rapid growth the patient requested biopsy.

During the second trimester in particular, the histology of these masses is characterized by large alveolar spaces filled with foamy material and cytoplasmic vacuoles. When these lesions undergo rapid growth, there may be infarction and necrosis, adding to the areas of cystic change seen on ultrasound. Generally, when the patient stops nursing or in the postpartum period, these lesions resolve or decrease significantly in size. However, during subsequent pregnancies, they may recur.

Notes

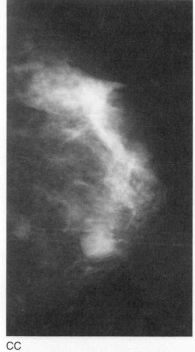

CC

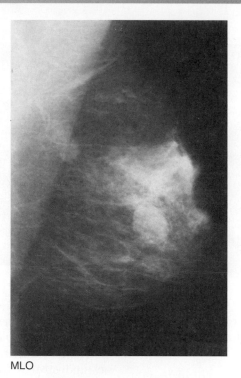

MLO

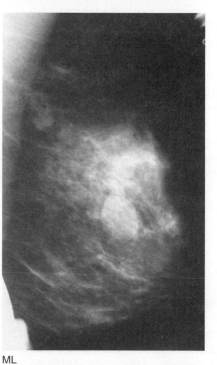

ML

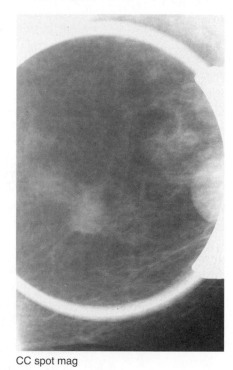

CC spot mag

1. There are two lesions in the right breast. Describe the anterior lesion and give a BI-RADS category.

2. Describe the more posterior lesion and give a BI-RADS category.

3. Predict the o'clock for the anterior lesion.

4. Predict the o'clock for the more posterior lesion. Why does the posterior lesion "move" more between the MLO and ML views than the anterior mass?

CASE 66

Cyst and Cancer Triangulation

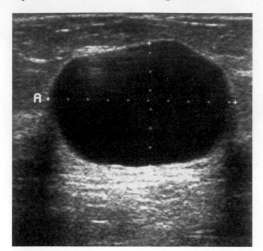

US anterior mass

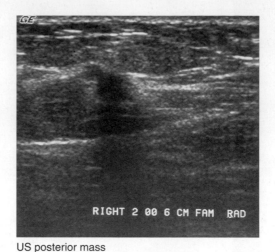

US posterior mass

1. There is an ovoid, partially circumscribed, high-density mass in the anterior medial breast. BI-RADS category 0: ultrasound is needed.

2. There is an irregular mass with possible spiculation in the upper inner breast. This should also be a BI-RADS category 0: both spot compression and ultrasound are needed.

3. The ovoid mass is at the 2 to 3 o'clock location, 2 cm from the areolar margin. Ultrasound reveals that this mass is a simple cyst—BI-RADS category 2: benign.

4. The posterior mass is high near the pectoralis muscle at 2 o'clock. This suspicious lesion is more peripheral in the breast and farther from the nipple; therefore, with changes in the projection angle (between MLO and ML), the mass moves more than the more anterior mass. Since this is a medial lesion, the lesion "moves up" from the MLO to the ML view. Ultrasound reveals that the mass has angular margins, is taller than wide, is very hypoechoic, and demonstrates posterior acoustic shadowing. This is a BI-RADS category 5: highly suspicious, biopsy is needed.

Reference

Stavros TA: *Breast Ultrasound*, Philadelphia, 2004, Lippincott Williams & Wilkins.

Cross-Reference

Ikeda, *Breast Imaging: THE REQUISITES*, p 47.

Comment

This case demonstrates an example of satisfaction of search. The ovoid mass seen in the anterior medial breast is immediately evident. Although mammographically the appearance suggests the benign etiology, such as a fibroadenoma or a cyst, because of the well-circumscribed margins, an ultrasound is necessary to determine whether it is cystic or solid. The optical density and size of the smooth round mass draw one's attention immediately and may distract one from carefully evaluating the remainder of the mammogram.

More posteriorly in the breast, there is a small irregular mass that could be missed if the reader's attention is on the more anterior round mass. Spot magnification views of the irregular mass show a suggestion of spiculation and faint calcifications. Ultrasound was performed not only to further characterize the mass but also to map out its location for potential biopsy under ultrasound guidance. The mass is seen on the initial cranial caudad view in the deep medial right breast. The MLO view shows the mass partially superimposed over the pectoralis muscle. The straight lateral view confirms that this is indeed the same mass because the mass is seen to "rise" or be more superiorly in the breast on the ML view. This moving of the mass "up" on the ML view is consistent with a medial lesion in the breast.

Ultrasound was performed deep along the upper inner breast at the 1 to 2 o'clock radius and the small, irregular, highly suspicious mass was visualized at the 2 o'clock site, 6 cm from the areolar margin while the patient was in the supine position. Sometimes, it is helpful to have patients sit up for imaging of ultrasound lesions in the high posterior breast. In this case, the patient should be positioned either flat on her back or possibly slightly rotated left anterior oblique so that the area of breast in which the suspicious lesion is thought to be located is optimally scanned.

Biopsy under ultrasound guidance of the irregular posterior mass revealed a 1-cm invasive ductal carcinoma. No intervention was needed for the anteriorly located cyst.

Notes

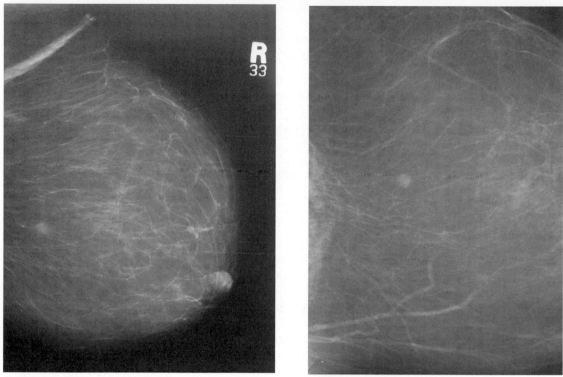

Cropped MLO view

Cropped CC view

1. An asymptomatic woman presents for a baseline screening mammogram. Based on the mammographic images, where do you think the right breast mass is located?

2. What clinical questions might you ask the patient when she returns for additional diagnostic imaging?

3. What additional mammographic view might you perform if there are pertinent clinical findings?

4. What ultrasound finding is pathognomonic for this benign condition?

Sebaceous Cyst

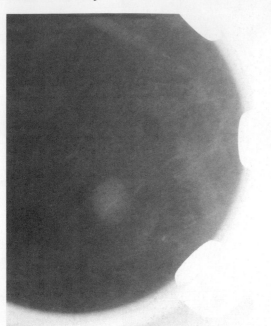

Spot mag CC view

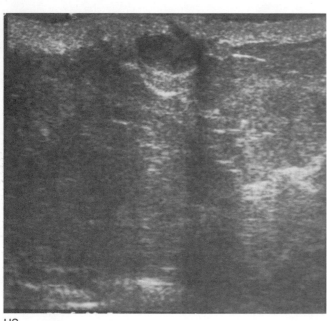

US

1. The position in the center of the breast on the CC view and in the inferior half of the breast on the MLO view suggests that the mass is probably at the 6 o'clock position.

2. The patient should be questioned about any areas of palpable concern and if there are any skin lesions or sebaceous cysts.

3. If there is a skin lesion, a metallic BB could be placed on the lesion and a repeat mammographic view performed.

4. The ultrasound finding of a thin neck extending to the skin from the very superficial hypoechoic mass is consistent with a benign sebaceous cyst.

Reference

Baker JA, Scott Soo M: Breast US: Assessment of technical quality and image interpretation, *Radiology* 223:229, 2002.

Cross-Reference

Ikeda, *Breast Imaging: THE REQUISITES*, p 128.

Comment

The mammographic views show an equal-density mass that triangulates to the inferior aspect of the breast. The position of the mass on the CC view is consistent with either a 12 or 6 o'clock location. The MLO confirms that the mass is in the inferior breast. Since the MLO is performed in the 45° angle, the mass does not appear at the inferior margin of the breast tissue. If a straight lateral view had been performed, the mass would be seen as very superficially located in the inferior breast. Questioning (and/or examination) of the patient may reveal an inflamed skin lesion consistent with a sebaceous cyst. Sebaceous cyst are retention cysts that originate in the sebaceous glands. They frequently occur in the inframammary fold along the inferior medial breast or in the periareolar location or axilla. Epidermal inclusion cysts are similar but arise with an obstructive hair follicle or in a traumatic skin disruption.

When there is a sebaceous cyst, a punctum, or black head, is often evident on physical exam. However, frequently, the patient is unaware of the sebaceous cyst because there is no superficial inflammation. In these cases, ultrasound may be particularly helpful. Ultrasound reveals a well-defined hypoechoic mass with a thin neck, which is the follicular duct extending through the echogenic skin layer to the skin surface. To image the neck, a standoff pad and a high-frequency transducer may be necessary. Once the etiology has been determined, no further evaluation is needed. Routine follow-up is adequate.

Notes

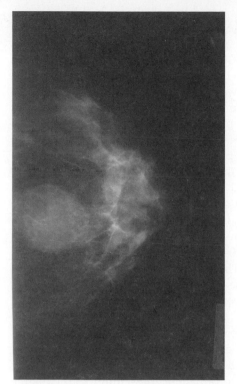

CC view

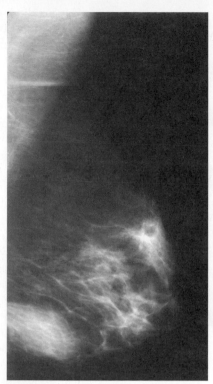

MLO

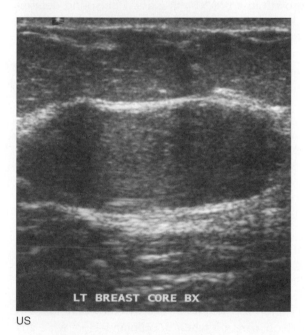

US

This 44-year-old woman presents with a rapidly growing mass in her inferior right breast.

1. Describe the mammographic and ultrasound findings.

2. What is the most likely diagnosis and what BI-RADS category would you give this?

3. The core biopsy yields "fibroepithelial lesion with high cellularity." What is the significance of this histology?

4. What is the appropriate management?

Benign Phyllodes Tumor

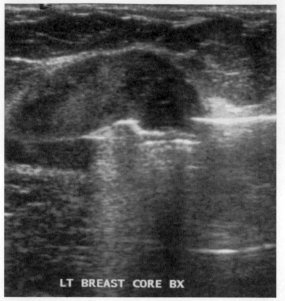

US guided biopsy

1. The mammogram shows a large equal-density ovoid mass with well-defined margins at the 6 o'clock site in the right breast. Ultrasound shows a large, hypoechoic, ovoid, solid mass with well-defined margins.

2. The most likely diagnosis is a benign fibroadenoma; however, core biopsy or excision are recommended because the lesion is large, newly palpable, and rapidly growing—BI-RADS category 4: lesion.

3. The histology on core was not definitive. This lesion could be a phyllodes tumor or a complex fibroadenoma.

4. Excisional biopsy is necessary because the diagnosis was not specific enough.

Reference

Liberman L, Bonaccio E, Hamele-Bena D, Abramson AF, Cohen MA, Dershaw DD: Benign and malignant phyllodes tumors: Mammographic and sonographic findings, *Radiology* 198:121, 1996.

Cross-Reference

Ikeda, *Breast Imaging: THE REQUISITES*, pp 110–113, 183.

Comment

Mammographically and on ultrasound, this lesion has a very benign appearance due to the ovoid, wider than tall shape and the sharp margins. However, the patient knew that the mass was new and growing, and she was concerned. Therefore, a biopsy was recommended.

If the patient had stated that the mass had been stable for many years and on breast exam the stability could be documented with prior mammograms or ultrasounds, a follow-up, rather than a biopsy, would suffice. On core biopsy, the lack of a definitive diagnosis of "fibroadenoma" was concerning. In addition, the high cellularity on core and the history of a rapid growth are concerning for a phyllodes tumor. Excision was recommended, and this was a benign phyllodes tumor.

Cystosarcoma phyllodes tumors account for approximately 0.3% of all breast tumors and usually occur as solitary, unilateral breast masses that tend, on average, to be larger than a fibroadenoma (many phyllodes are larger than 4 cm). In addition, the average age of patients with phyllodes tumors is approximately 45 years, or approximately 10–15 years older than patients with fibroadenomas. The tumors are thought to be hormonally responsive, as are fibroadenomas.

Mammographically, the masses are usually dense, oval or round, noncalcified, smoothly marginated masses that appear almost identical to fibroadenomas but rarely have calcifications. Approximately 20% of cases are detected as nonpalpable masses on screening mammograms, and of patients presenting with palpable lesions, approximately 20–30% give a history of sudden rapid growth in a preexistent mass. Ultrasound demonstrates hypoechoic, isoechoic, or even heterogeneous masses that often have irregular cystic spaces.

Histologically, the tumors are composed of cellular spindle cell fibroblasts with leaflike (hence, "phyllodes") processes that protrude into cystic spaces. The staging or grading of the phyllodes is dependent on the margin and cell types seen histologically. There may be highly atypical or multinucleated giant cells; low-grade phyllodes have pushing margins with mild atypia. High-grade or infiltrative margins have moderate to severe atypia, and surgical excision with a margin greater than 1 cm is recommend. Five-year survival for the malignant form is 55–75%.

The most common diagnostic problem is distinguishing from a core biopsy specimen which lesions are histologically benign or borderline phyllodes tumors and which lesions are the more common fibroadenomas. Because of sampling issues, this is not always possible. Therefore, when a nonspecific diagnosis is obtained on core or when a cellular lesion with any form of spindle cells is seen, excision is recommended.

Notes

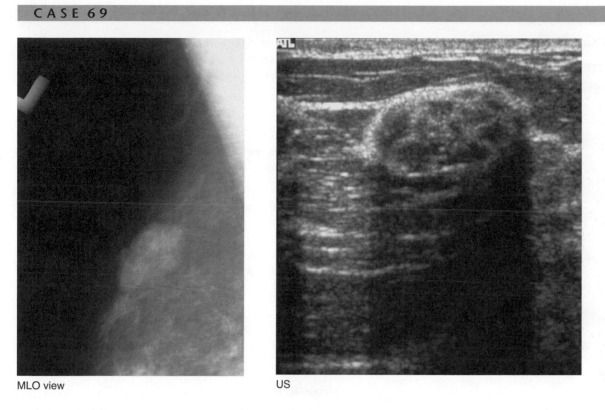

MLO view   US

A 41-year-old woman presents with a palpable mass in the upper left breast.

1. Describe the mammographic findings.

2. Describe the ultrasound findings.

3. What is the likelihood of malignancy? Does the lesion need to be biopsied?

4. The biopsy results yielded a "complex fibroadenoma." Describe the clinical significance of these results.

Complex Fibroadenoma

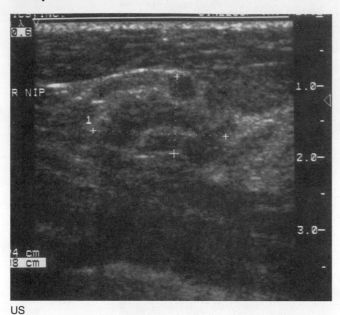

US

1. The mammogram shows a well-defined, equal-density, ovoid mass in the upper left breast. Ultrasound is useful for further characterization.

2. The ultrasound shows a heterogeneous solid mass with a complex internal structure and microlobulated margins.

3. Biopsy is recommended; however, this most likely represents a fibroadenoma.

4. Complex fibroadenoma is a diagnosis that may be obtained from a core biopsy. This histology does not require excision if there is no atypia present. However, the diagnosis of a complex fibroadenoma is associated with an increased risk for subsequent development of breast cancer in this patient.

Reference

DuPont WD, Page DL, Pari FF, et al.: Long term risk of breast cancer in women with fibroadenoma, *N Engl J Med* 351(1):10–15, 1994.

Cross-Reference

Ikeda, *Breast Imaging: THE REQUISITES*, pp 110, 141.

Comment

The term *complex fibroadenoma* describes a fibroadenoma that contains proliferative changes, such as sclerosing adenosis, ductal hyperplasia, or papillary apocrine metaplasia (cyst formation). Dupont et al. coined the term and found that approximately 33% of fibroadenomas could be classified as "complex" based on the histologic findings. They found that these lesions were associated with an increased risk for subsequent development of breast cancer at a rate approximately 3.88 times that of the normal population. Although excision is not necessary, it is important to educate patients with any type of histologic "risk" lesion that they have a higher than average risk of developing breast cancer in the future. It is important to understand that the complex fibroadenoma and the proliferative changes that characterize the lesion are markers of risk for both breasts. It is very unlikely that a cancer would arise within the complex fibroadenoma, but the proliferative changes found on biopsy are indicative of diffuse proliferative changes in the breasts bilaterally.

Notes

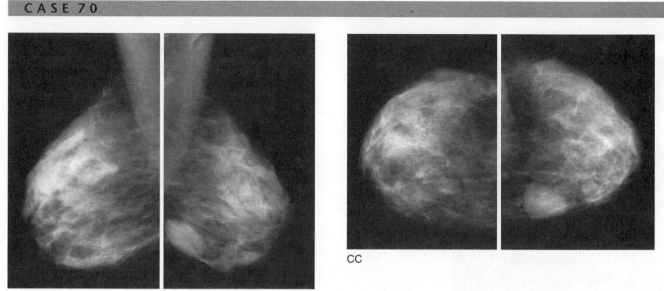

MLO

CC

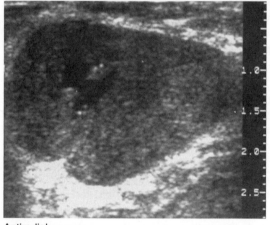

Antiradial

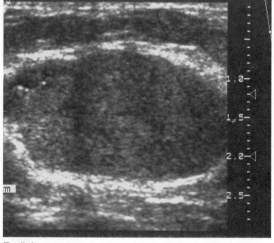

Radial

This 35-year-old woman presents with a rapidly growing right breast mass. She had a renal transplant 3 years ago and is on cyclosporin A therapy.

1. Describe the mammographic findings.

2. Describe the ultrasound findings.

3. What is the most likely diagnosis and etiology of the lesion?

4. Is biopsy necessary?

Cyclosporin-Induced Fibroadenoma

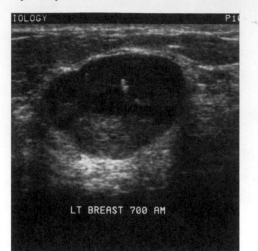

LT BREAST 700 AM

1. There is a well-circumscribed, high-density mass in the inferior medial right breast.

2. The macrolobulated solid mass is well circumscribed and has internal cystic areas.

3. The history hints that the patient may be on cyclosporin A for her renal transplant. If so, the most likely diagnosis is a cyclosporin-induced fibroadenoma.

4. Yes, but core biopsy is adequate to confirm the benign etiology of this large, rapidly growing mass.

Reference

Weinstein SP, Orel SG, Collazzo L, Conant EF, Lawton TJ, Czerniecki B: Cyclosporin A–induced fibroadenomas of the breast: Report of five cases. *Radiology* 220(2):465–468, 2001.

Cross-Reference

Ikeda, *Breast Imaging: THE REQUISITES*, p 110.

Comment

The mammogram reveals a large ovoid solid mass with well-circumscribed margins. Ultrasound reveals that there are internal cystic spaces that may be seen in both benign fibroadenomas and also the rare phyllodes tumor. The clinical history of cyclosporin use and the mammographic and ultrasound findings are most consistent with a benign fibroadenoma. However, since the mass was rapidly growing, a biopsy was recommended. The biopsy confirms the benign diagnosis of a fibroadenoma.

Fibroadenomas have been described as a sequelae of cyclosporin A therapy, particularly in patients on the medication following renal transplantation. The exact mechanism for the induction of the often bilateral and multiple large fibroadenomas is not entirely known. Various mechanisms have been suggested, including the effect of cyclosporin on fibroblasts (some fibroblasts have cyclosporin receptors) and the effect that cyclosporin has on the hypothalamic–pituitary axis. An alternative mechanism involves antagonism of the prolactin receptor sites on B and T lymphocytes by cyclosporin A. It has been noted that the use of cyclosporin A may result in elevated prolactin levels, which may have a direct tropic effect on the fibroblasts in fibroadenomas. In one study, the duration of cyclosporin A therapy in patients in whom fibroadenomas were diagnosed ranged from 23 to 126 months. It has also been noted that when cyclosporin is withdrawn, the fibroadenomas may resolve.

Notes

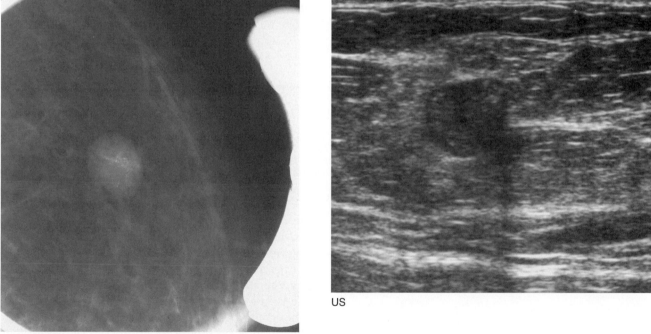

MLO

CC

Spot mag CC

US

1. There is a mass in the upper right breast that had remained stable in size for many years. However, on the screening mammogram, the mass has developed faint calcifications. What is the most likely diagnosis for this mass?

2. What BI-RADS category should be used?

3. Does the ultrasound help determine if this is a lymph node?

4. What type of biopsy should be done?

Complex Fibroadenoma/DCIS

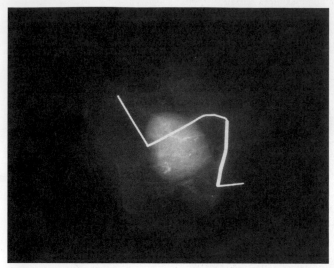

Specimen radiograph

1. The most likely diagnosis is a fibroadenoma, perhaps of the complex subtype because of the calcifications or, less likely, a lymph node. However, the change over time with the appearance of new calcifications in the mass is concerning.

2. A BI-RADS category 0 should initially be given and the patient should be called back for magnification views of the calcifications. Magnification views reveal that the calcifications are heterogeneous or pleomorphic, and a biopsy is recommended.

3. The mass does not have the typical echogenic fatty hilum that should be seen in a lymph node on ultrasound. The mass has fairly well-circumscribed but suspicious pleomorphic calcifications that are seen on both mammography and ultrasound, raising the concern that this is at least a complex fibroadenoma. Biopsy is recommended.

4. In this case, excision was recommended because there was a high likelihood that the faint calcifications would be at least due to atypical ductal hyperplasia. On excision, this lesion had DCIS within the complex fibroadenoma.

Reference

DuPont WD, Page DL, Pari FF, et al.: Long term risk of breast cancer in women with fibroadenoma, *N Engl J Med* 351(1):10–15, 1994.

Cross-Reference

Ikeda, *Breast Imaging: THE REQUISITES*, pp 110, 141.

Comment

This is a somewhat unusual case of a complex fibroadenoma (CFA) that develops DCIS. Presumably, this CFA had ductal proliferative carcinoma that progressed to DCIS. Thirty-three percent of fibroadenomas are thought to be classifiable as "complex" based on the superimposed fibrocystic changes, cyst larger than 3 mm, sclerosing adenosis, epithelial calcifications, and papillary apocrine changes seen in the stroma. The more severe the proliferative changes, the higher the risk for developing breast cancer in an individual patient. The CFAs are thought to be a marker for increased risk only when proliferation is present. Therefore, core biopsy is adequate for diagnosis if there is no atypia. In this case, the calcifications were new and pleomorphic, and therefore an excision was recommended rather than a core. DCIS was found within the ductal elements in the fibroadenoma.

Notes

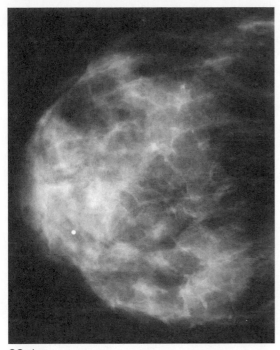

CC view

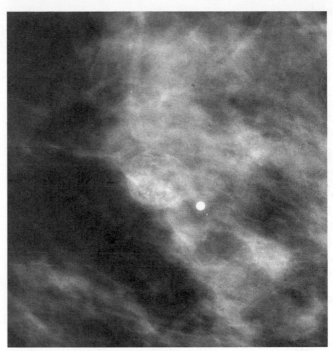

Mag view CC

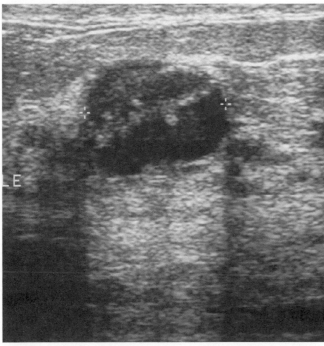

US

1. This 34-year-old woman presents with a small palpable mass in the left breast. She gives a history of stopping nursing approximately 3 months previously. How does the workup for this patient begin?

2. Describe the mammographic findings best seen on the magnified CC view of the area under the metallic BB.

3. Describe the ultrasound findings.

4. What is the most likely diagnosis and what BI-RADS category should be used?

Galactocele

1. Since the patient is older than 30 years of age, the workup began with a mammogram. A metallic BB was placed on the area of palpable concern in the left breast.

2. A mixed-density (area of lucency and soft tissue density), very well-circumscribed mass is seen underlying the metallic BB on the spot magnification view.

3. On ultrasound, the mass has a complex layered appearance with echogenic material anteriorly.

4. Given the patient's history of recent lactation and the benign-appearing imaging findings, the most likely diagnosis is a galactocele. This is a BI-RADS category 2: benign. Routine follow-up is recommended.

Reference

Berg WA, Campassi CI, Ioffe OB: Cystic lesions of the breast: Sonographic-pathologic correlation, *Radiology* 227:183, 2003.

Cross-Reference

Ikeda, *Breast Imaging: THE REQUISITES*, p 128.

Comment

The most likely diagnosis for this complex cystic mass is a galactocele in this patient, who has recently stopped nursing. Since the patient is older than 30 years of age, mammography is the first study of choice. A small radiolucent mass is present in the area of palpable concern, as marked by the metallic BB. The ultrasound was performed to directly correlate the physical findings with the mammographic findings and to exclude any suspicious ultrasound findings. The mammographic and ultrasound findings are concordant, and both are consistent with a benign galactocele, a benign cystic space filled with milk products, presumably caused by some form of ductal obstruction. Galactoceles usually present as palpable, nontender masses during lactation or within a few months after cessation of lactation.

The mammographic and ultrasound findings vary depending on the amount of fat and proteinaceous material in a galactocele. In this case, the galactocele is more mature and is almost entirely filled with fatty material making it partially lucent on mammography, similar to the appearance of an oil cyst. Ultrasound findings may vary as well, from circumscribed masses with fluid debris levels to solid-appearing masses with very low-level internal echoes. In this case, the fatty contents of the galactocele are in the superior portion as the more echogenic material in the mass. The mammographic appearance of a mixed-density mass (partially lucent)

and the ultrasound appearance of a mixed-echotecture complex cystic mass are very similar to fat necrosis, which should be included in the differential diagnosis. No intervention is needed when the imaging findings are correlated carefully with the history and physical exam.

Notes

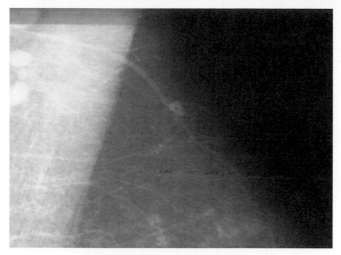

Initial cropped MLO

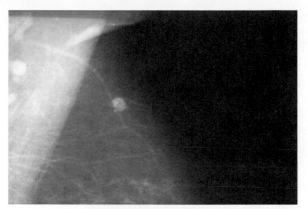

2 years later, cropped MLO

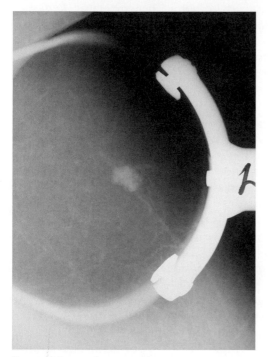

2 years later, spot compression

1. What is the change in the right MLO view between the initial image and two years later?

2. What is in your differential diagnosis for this unilateral finding?

3. What additional imaging would you perform?

4. Would you biopsy this lesion?

Lymphoma in Intramammary Node

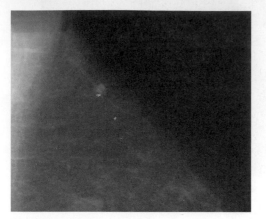

Post biopsy with clip

1. The low-lying right axillary node has enlarged, become increasingly dense, and has lost its fatty hilum.

2. Malignancy from breast, melanoma, or lymphoma. Benign hypertrophy, inflammatory, and infectious causes are less likely.

3. Ultrasound would be helpful to further characterize the lesion and guide future biopsy.

4. Biopsy, ideally with needle core technique, is a useful next step.

References

Cyrlak D, Carpenter PM: Cases of the day: Breast imaging case of the day, *RadioGraphics* 19:S73–S79, 1999.

Lee CH, Giurescu ME, Philpotts LE, Horvath LJ, Tocino I: Clinical importance of unilaterally enlarging lymph nodes on otherwise normal mammograms, *Radiology* 203:329–334, 1997.

Cross-Reference

Ikeda, *Breast Imaging: THE REQUISITES*, p 117.

Comment

In this 68-year-old woman, a right intramammary node was noted to have enlarged on her screening mammogram compared to the prior exam. On the earlier exam, the right lymph node can be seen to be oval in shape, has a low density, and contains a fatty hilum. The cortex is symmetric. These are features of a normal lymph node. No further imaging is needed. However, on the following mammogram 2 years later, this node is denser and has irregular margins. The previously seen architecture of a normal node is no longer seen, and the node has increased in size and has lost its fatty hilum.

This change in a solitary, unilateral node may be due to benign causes, such as granulomatous disease, collagen vascular disease, infection, or hyperplasia, but metastatic disease and lymphoma must be considered first. Metastatic disease could develop in the node from a breast, lung, or melanoma primary. Needle core biopsy of the node will give the histology of the disease causing the enlargement, and it can help tailor the remaining workup.

If the node contains metastatic breast cancer and no primary malignancy is seen on mammogram, MRI is used to evaluate for occult cancer because it has a higher sensitivity for invasive tumor than mammography and ultrasound.

This patient underwent an ultrasound-guided needle core biopsy that showed grade I follicular lymphoma. A clip was placed after the biopsy to document the location and to mark the lesion in case surgery is needed.

Notes

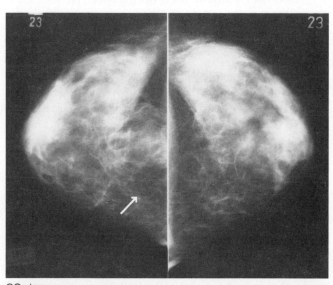

CC views

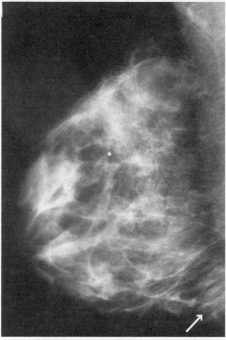

Left MLO

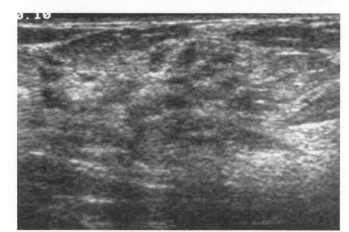

US at 6:00

This patient had recently started on hormone replacement therapy and presented with a newly palpable area of "thickening" interiorly in the left breast.

1. Describe the mammographic finding in the left breast, best seen posteriorly and centrally on the CC view.

2. Where is the finding on the MLO view?

3. Describe any findings on the ultrasound.

4. Is any further imaging needed? What is the most likely diagnosis?

Accessory Breast Tissue

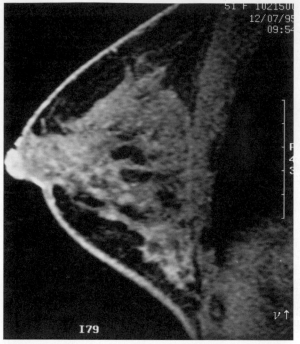

MRI post Gd

1. There is a focal asymmetry in the posterior central left breast. The asymmetry has a mixed density.

2. The focal asymmetry is in the very inferior left breast, only partially seen on the MLO view.

3. Ultrasound shows what appears to be normal glandular and ductal tissue without evidence of a suspicious mass.

4. No further imaging is needed; however, the patient was referred for a MRI by her physician because the area was newly palpable. The images are shown here. There is a good correlation in location and appearance on the MRI of normal accessory breast tissue along the inferior aspect of the "milk line."

Reference

Dixon JM, Mansel RE: ABC of breast diseases: Congenital problems and aberrations of normal breast development and involution, *Br Med J* 309:797–800, 1994.

Cross-Reference

Ikeda, *Breast Imaging: THE REQUISITES*, p 37.

Comment

Accessory breast tissue is found in approximately 2–6% of women. Most often, the tissue is found in the axillary region of the breast, arising in the tail of Spence or axillary tail breast tissue. Less common is accessory breast tissue along the inferior portion of the milk line, which extends from the central and inferior portion of the breast down to the groin. Incomplete regression or remnants of the primitive milk line may lead to accessory mounds or supernumerary nipples along the milk line.

On physical exam, these areas of accessory tissue may present as focal mounds or areas of thickening. On mammography, a nonspecific area of mixed fatty and glandular density may be seen, and occasionally a nipple may be seen on tangential views of the skin. Ultrasound will show the normal architecture of fat lobules and glandular and ductal elements and may be very useful to exclude a focal mass when the mound of ectopic tissue is pronounced and palpable. Generally, ultrasound and physical exam are sufficient to establish the diagnosis of normal accessory tissue, but in this case the area was newly palpable and as an alternative to biopsy, a MRI was performed. The area of ectopic breast tissue was easily identified inferiorly in the breast. The signal and enhancement pattern was that of normal glandular tissue, which further supported the benign diagnosis. Routine follow-up was recommended.

Notes

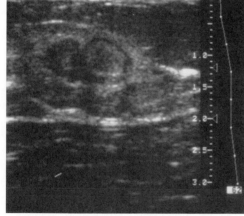

MLO view

Mag view

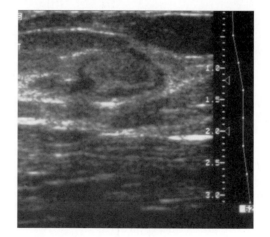

US

1. Describe the mammographic findings in this patient with a new palpable breast mass.

2. Describe the ultrasound findings and give a differential diagnosis.

3. What pertinent questions might you ask a patient regarding the clinical history and what might you look for on physical exam?

4. What final BI-RADS assessment category and specific follow-up recommendations are appropriate?

Hematoma of the Breast

1. The mammographic finding is a "focal asymmetry" of mixed density. (This finding is not a mammographic mass since it lacks distinct convex borders.)

2. On ultrasound, there is a mixed-echotecture mass in the breast that corresponds to the area of palpable concern and the area seen on the mammogram. The central area is hypoechoic and almost cystic, but the area is much larger, as shown by the echogenic material tracking along the Cooper's ligament into the surrounding tissue. The combination of the mixed-density focal asymmetry on mammography and the appearance on ultrasound is consistent with a hematoma.

3. The patient should be questioned regarding recent trauma. The breast should also be examined for any signs of bruising.

4. A BI-RADS 2: benign, if the clinical history is appropriate. However, if there is concern regarding the history or lack of history and the imaging findings, a category 3 with short-term follow-up in 6–8 weeks should be considered.

Cross-Reference

Ikeda, *Breast Imaging: THE REQUISITES*, p 124.

Comment

The appearance of a poorly defined but mixed-density focal asymmetry should evoke a differential diagnosis that includes hematoma and, of course, cancer. Generally, if patients are carefully questioned they are able to remember if there has been a traumatic incident to the breast. Occasionally, patients do not recall any recent trauma. The palpable component of the hematoma may actually occur weeks after visible bruising from the breast trauma as the hematoma matures and coalesces, becoming firmer on breast exam.

Mammographically, an early hematoma may have poorly defined margins, with high-density material (blood) tracking along the Cooper's ligaments into the surrounding tissue often appearing as an echogenic halo. There is rarely any distortion. Depending on the severity of the hematoma, the central area may be denser and even masslike due to the collection of blood. As the hematoma becomes better organized (and firmer on exam), the density may coalesce. Later changes may include slight distortion or even the development of fat necrosis. As the lesion is followed over time, the size should decrease and there should be complete resolution or the appearance of the typical changes of fat necrosis.

The ultrasound appearance may be quite confusing. Frequently, ultrasound reveals a mixed-echo area larger than that recognized mammographically. A large hematoma may have loculated areas with large septations seen on ultrasound, similar to the appearance of a seroma. Over time, the area may be better defined and become more hypoechoic and then resolve. If there is any suspicious area or lack of convincing history, short-term follow-up is recommended to exclude an underlying small malignancy that bled.

Notes

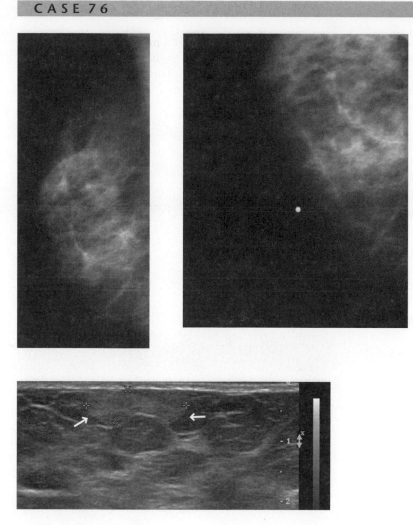

1. This patient feels a lump in the left breast. How should the technologist note the area of concern?

2. The marker overlies fat on the mammogram. Is there need for additional workup?

3. There is a hyperechoic mass seen on ultrasound. Is this finding suspicious?

4. Are there any malignant lesions that may appear hyperechoic on ultrasound of the breast?

Lipoma

1. A metal BB marker should be placed on the area of the patient's concern by the technologist before the bilateral mammogram is done, and the area of palpable concern should be noted on the patient information sheet.

2. Spot compression view of the patient's area of concern can be performed. Ultrasound is also necessary, along with a clinical exam of the area of concern.

3. The mass is completely hyperechoic and is oval, wider than tall, and gently lobulated—all benign features.

4. A tiny malignant mass can have a thick hyperechoic rim, possibly indicating desmoplastic reaction or infiltrative margin. A careful search should be made for a hypoechoic mass inside a hyperechoic one, especially if the mass is round, irregular, or vertically oriented.

Reference

Stavros AT: *Breast Ultrasound*, Philadelphia, 2004, Lippincott Williams & Wilkins, p 569.

Cross-Reference

Ikeda, *Breast Imaging: THE REQUISITES*, p 122.

Comment

This patient presents with a palpable finding and a negative mammogram. The value of ultrasound in this situation is clear. The palpable finding may be normal glandular tissue, a cyst, or a solid mass. The solid mass may have benign characteristics, indeterminate characteristics, or suspicious characteristics. The decision as to management depends on the nature of the ultrasound appearance.

In this case, the mass is well defined, horizontally aligned (wider than tall), purely echogenic, which are features of a benign mass, most likely a lipoma. Lipomas are benign overgrowths of adipose tissue, and the palpable lipomas are most commonly seen in subcutaneous fat. They may develop fat necrosis but only rarely develop sarcomatous changes. They are seen as commonly in men as in women, and they occur throughout the body.

Ultrasound features of lipomas include those isoechoic or hyperechoic to the surrounding fat. The mass may be seen on the mammogram as an area of fat lucency, but characteristically it is not identified on mammography because it cannot be distinguished from radiolucent fat.

This patient can be reassured that no biopsy is needed. She can be placed into routine follow-up care.

Notes

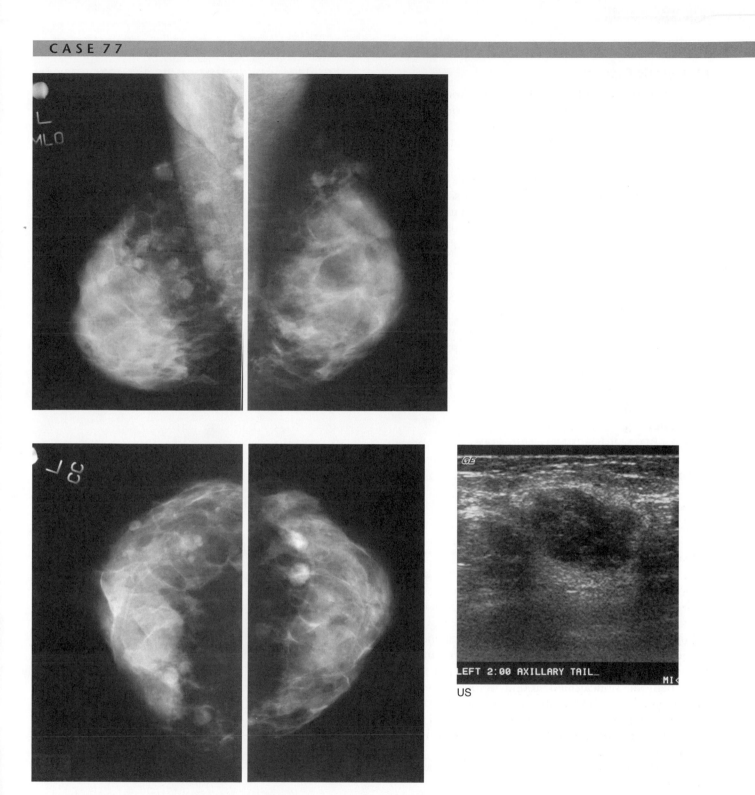

US

1. A 43-year-old presents with multiple bilateral breast lumps and subcutaneous nodules. What clinical questions might you ask?

2. Describe the mammographic and ultrasound findings.

3. Give the differential diagnosis of multiple solid breast masses.

4. What is the appropriate management?

Metastatic Disease

1. A general medical history should be taken with important questions including the following: Has this patient ever had prior breast masses biopsied? Does the patient have any known malignancies?

2. The patient has multiple bilateral breast masses that on mammography have partially defined margins and on ultrasound are hypoechoic and solid. Some of the breast masses are actually subcutaneous nodules. The margins of the masses on ultrasound are poorly defined and there are microlobulations. The ultrasound appearance is more concerning than the mammographic appearance.

3. Although fibroadenomas and papillomas may be multiple and bilateral, the appearance of these masses and the history of subcutaneous nodules are more concerning for diffuse metastases.

4. Biopsy was recommended and was performed as a core biopsy under ultrasound guidance.

Reference

Toombs BD, Kalisher L: Metastatic disease in the breast: Clinical, pathologic, and radiographic features, *Am J Roentgenol* 129:673–676, 1977.

Cross-Reference

Ikeda, *Breast Imaging: THE REQUISITES*, p 109.

Comment

The patient has multiple masses in both breasts. Although this mammographic appearance may be seen with multiple fibroadenomas or papillomas, the hypoechoic and poorly defined masses that lack a thin echogenic rim on ultrasound have an appearance that suggests a more ominous etiology, such as multiple metastases. In general, metastases to the breast tend to be superficial, noncalcified, round or oval masses on mammography with partially circumscribed or fading margins. Ultrasound often reveals hypoechoic solid masses with well-defined or poorly defined margins that are often quite vascular. Careful questioning of the patient is recommended so that if the patient has a known primary malignancy, biopsy may not be necessary.

In this case, the patient had no known primary malignancy, and core biopsy of one of the larger masses was performed with ultrasound guidance. Adenocarcinoma was obtained. The patient went on to have an abdominal CT that showed extensive liver metastases. No primary malignancy was ever found.

Breast-to-breast metastases are the most common metastatic lesions involving the breast. Extramammary metastases represent approximately 1% of all breast malignancies. In this case, the masses are innumerable and there is no history of primary breast carcinoma, so an extramammary source must be searched for. Lymphomas and leukemias are the most common metastases to involve the breast, followed by metastases from melanoma, lung, prostate, ovary, gastrointestinal malignancies, and cervical cancers.

Notes

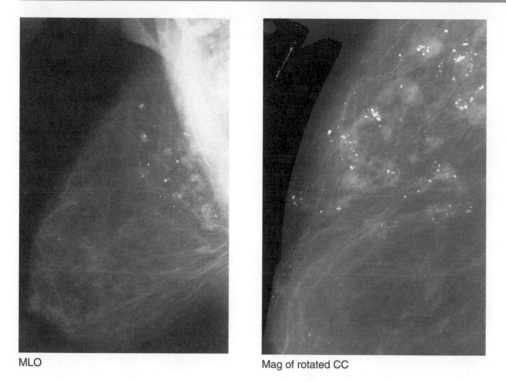

MLO

Mag of rotated CC

1. Describe the unilateral findings in this baseline screening mammogram in a 63-year-old woman.

2. What is the BI-RADS category and recommendation?

3. What is the differential diagnosis?

4. Biopsy reveals granulomatous changes with acid-fast organisms seen on special stains. What additional imaging study might be helpful?

Tuberculosis Nodes

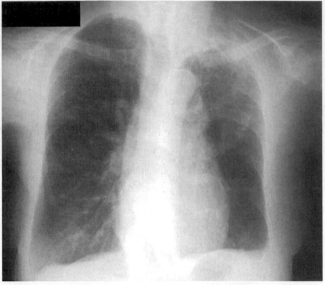

CXR

1. There are extensive calcifications in the axillary tail of the left breast.

2. A BI-RADS category 0: incomplete, additional imaging is needed. The patient should be called back for magnification views of the calcifications.

3. Magnification performed with lateral exaggeration in the cranial caudad view shows that there are clustered heterogeneous calcifications associated with nodules in the axillary tail of the breast. Some of the larger calcifications may be due to fat necrosis, but there are fainter, more concerning heterogeneous calcifications. The nodular pattern in the axillary tail may be due to trauma or an inflammatory process, but the faint calcifications prompted the recommendation for a biopsy.

4. The next imaging study should be a chest x-ray. This patient had tuberculous changes on the chest x-ray, and changes in the left axilla were due to extension of the infection into the axilla and lateral breast.

Cross-Reference
Ikeda, *Breast Imaging: THE REQUISITES*, p 71.

Comment
The calcifications that are in the right axilla have a very unusual appearance. Although some of the calcifications appear to be coarse and benign, there are fainter calcifications extending into the low axilla. The multiple nodules are difficult to discern but may represent small masses and possibly lymph nodes in the axillary tail of the breast. On biopsy, the calcifications were due to a granulomatous process associated with caseating granulomas. These findings are consistent with tuberculosis, and acid-fast organisms were seen on special stains. A chest x-ray shows that there is left apical capping and calcifications typical of tuberculous changes in the lung. In this case, the patient had a tuberculous infection similar to scrofula of the neck, but instead of extending up into the soft tissues of the neck, the granulomatous changes extended into the axilla. The findings are all benign, but a biopsy was necessary to exclude malignancy because of the heterogeneous nature of some of the calcifications.

This case demonstrates that findings on a mammogram may be indicative of a more system process, in this case, a granulomatous infection. Careful questioning of the patient is essential so that breast imaging findings can be incorporated in the more global care of the patient. In this case, if the radiologist had known of the extensive granulomatous changes in the left chest and axilla, a breast biopsy could have been avoided.

Notes

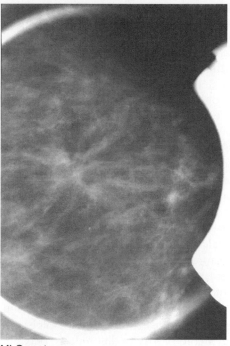

MLO spot mag

1. This 45-year-old woman presents with a very subtle area of architectural distortion that may have been present on the past three prior mammographic studies. What is the differential diagnosis for this lesion?

2. What is the BI-RADS category and recommendation?

3. Core biopsy was performed and elongated tubules were seen in this small invasive ductal carcinoma. What histologic subtype is this, most likely?

4. What is the prognosis?

Tubular Cancer

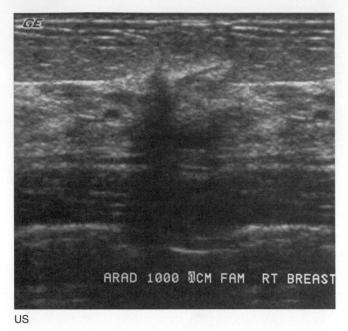

US

1. The differential diagnosis includes invasive ductal carcinoma not otherwise specified, tubular carcinoma, and a radial sclerosing lesion.

2. Category 4: suspicious, biopsy recommended.

3. The elongated tubules seen histologically suggest the tubular subtype of invasive ductal carcinoma.

4. The prognosis for these well-differentiated cancers is better than that for not otherwise specified invasive ductal carcinoma.

Reference

Feig SA, Shaber GS, Patchefsky AS, Schwartz GF, Edeiken J, Nerlinger R: Tubular carcinoma of the breast: Mammographic appearance and pathological correlation, *Radiology* 129:311, 1978.

Cross-Reference

Ikeda, *Breast Imaging: THE REQUISITES*, pp 98–99.

Comment

Tubular carcinomas are uncommon breast cancers, comprising less than 2% of all breast cancers. They tend to be very well differentiated and have a very slow growth rate. Mammographically, they are small spiculated masses or areas of architectural distortion. If a spiculated mass is seen, the arms of the spicules often extend for a distance longer than the size of the central mass. These often subtle cancers may be difficult to differentiate from radial scars or small invasive ductal carcinomas. Amorphous microcalcifications occur in approximately 10–15% of cases. On ultrasound, these subtle lesions may be difficult to see. Often, there is only subtle distortion that may be seen in only one plane of scanning. This is due to the fact that, as on mammography and histologically, architectural distortion is the most impressive feature; there is often very little, if any, central tumor mass.

Pathologically, the invasive tumor cells form angulated tubular glands that are surrounded by a desmoplastic reaction of stromal elastosis. Tubular carcinomas may sometimes be confused with benign proliferative lesions, such as radial sclerosing lesions and florid sclerosing adenosis, particularly when the carcinoma is associated with amorphous calcifications. However, the distinguishing pathologic features include a single layer of cells lining the tubules and loss of the lobular architecture with infiltration into the surrounding tissues. The benign proliferative lesions are characterized by glands with double cell layers. Pathologists may need an excisional biopsy rather than a core biopsy to differentiate between the benign and the malignant lesions if the double cell layer is not clearly seen in sampling.

Tubular carcinomas may have mixed forms, but the pure form of tubular carcinoma is associated with an excellent prognosis. Only approximately 10% of patients have axillary metastases at the time of diagnosis. As can be expected, as the percentage of not otherwise specified invasive ductal carcinoma associated with the tubular carcinoma increases, there is a higher incidence of metastases.

Notes

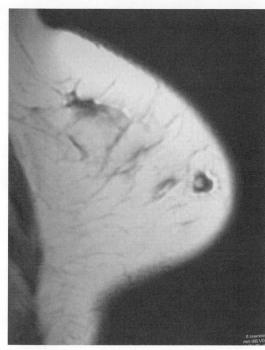

T1 weighted

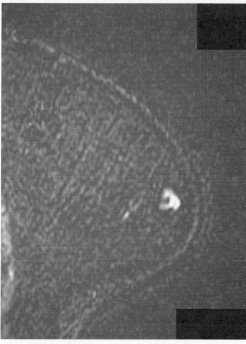

MR subtraction

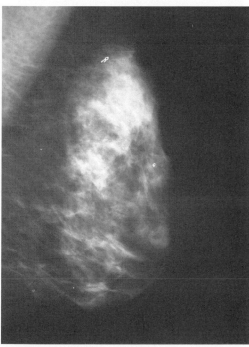

MLO view

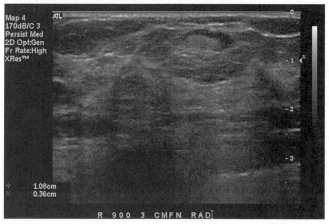

US

1. Describe the MRI findings.

2. What is the most likely diagnosis?

3. Does ultrasound help in this evaluation?

4. The MRI was requested because she has a history of malignancy in the other breast. Is this an acceptable use of MRI?

MRI, Mammography, and Ultrasound of Normal Intramammary Lymph Node

1. There is an enhancing mass in the right anterior breast, containing fat on T1.

2. This is consistent with an intramammary lymph node.

3. Ultrasound is not necessary in this case since the MRI findings are pathognomonic. US is helpful as a targeted exam after equivocal findings are seen on MRI.

4. Yes, MRI is used to evaluate the ipsilateral and contralateral breasts after a diagnosis of breast cancer.

References

LaTrenta LR, Menell JH, Morris EA, Abramson AF, Dershaw DD, Liberman L: Breast lesions detected with MR imaging: Utility and histopathologic importance of identification with US, *Radiology* 227(3):856–861, 2003.

Teifke A, Lehr HA, Vomweg TW, Hlawatsch A, Thelen M: Outcome analysis and rational management of enhancing lesions incidentally detected on contrast-enhanced MRI of the breast, *Am J Roentgenol* 181(3):655–662, 2003.

Cross-Reference

Ikeda, *Breast Imaging: THE REQUISITES*, p 205.

Comment

This is a 66-year-old patient who has a recent history of left breast cancer. She underwent breast MRI for high-risk screening. This is a useful indication for breast MRI, particularly in the patient with a mammographically dense breast.

The MR images shown are a subtraction image and a T1-weighted image. The images demonstrate a well-defined enhancing mass that contains a central fatty hilum. Fat-containing masses in the breast are generally benign. This lymph node is relatively close to the nipple and is 11 mm in length—a somewhat unusual location and size. Typically, intramammary lymph nodes are located in the upper outer quadrant and are smaller than 5 mm.

The mammogram should be reviewed when interpreting breast MRI. In this patient, there is a fat-containing lymph node in the anterior right breast, which is stable in size on mammograms dating back several years, corresponding in location and size to the MRI finding. Because of the stability and normal appearance of this node, no further evaluation is needed.

Notes

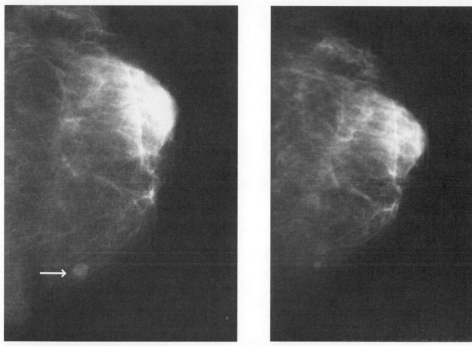

Initial mammogram, CC view

2-month follow-up, CC view

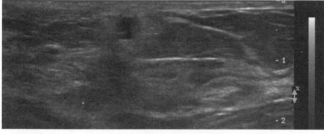

Initial US

1. The arrow is pointing to the area of palpable concern. Describe the finding.

2. The patient reports trauma from seat belt injury, with bruising over the medial right breast. Is the density related?

3. What is the differential diagnosis for this developing mass (new since previous mammogram)?

4. What should be done next to narrow the diagnosis?

Hematoma

1. There is a sharply circumscribed, moderate-density, round mass in the medial right breast.

2. The mass is at the site of trauma; it may be related.

3. The differential diagnosis includes benign and malignant masses, a cyst, and a hematoma.

4. Ultrasound is important to help differentiate masses, cysts, and hematoma.

References

Kanegusuku MS, Rodrigues D, Dirceu U, et al.: Recurrent spontaneous breast hematoma: Report of a case and review of the literature, *Rev Hosp Clin* 56(6):179–182, 2001.

Mendelson EB: Evaluation of the postoperative breast, *Radiol Clin North Am* 30(1):107–138, 1992.

Cross-Reference

Ikeda, *Breast Imaging: THE REQUISITES*, p 124.

Comment

This patient presented for a routine mammogram, and a new mass was seen in the medial lower right breast. This mass is round, sharply circumscribed, and of moderate density. There was bruising in the medial right breast, and the patient reported that a motor vehicle accident had occurred several weeks before. The bruising at that time had been in the medial right breast, where the seat belt crossed her chest. The area of new mass on the mammogram was in the area of the bruising.

Ultrasound shows a hypoechoic mass with echogenic rim, which is consistent with hematoma. The mass is seen in the area of bruising. A malignant mass may have an identical ultrasound appearance. An occult cancer can present after trauma because of bleeding into the malignant mass.

In order to confirm the diagnosis of hematoma due to seat belt injury, a short-term follow-up is recommended, with a follow-up unilateral mammogram in 6–8 weeks.

The patient was asked to return in 2 months. Her right mammogram after 2 months shows that the mass has decreased in size, consistent with healing. However, the area must be followed to complete resolution to confirm the benign etiology. The time of resolution of a hematoma is variable and may depend on patient age as well as severity of the injury.

Notes

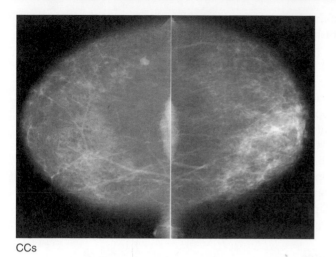

CCs

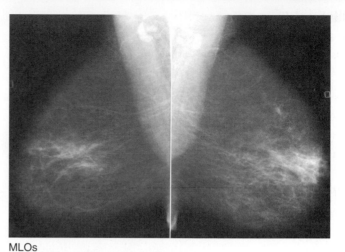

MLOs

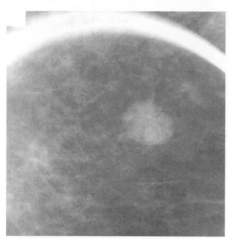

Left CC spot

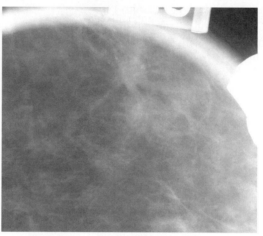

Right CC spot

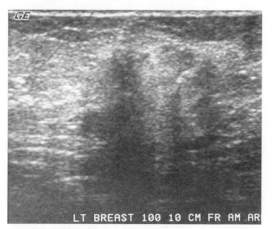

Left US

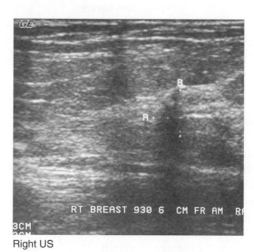

Right US

1. Define synchronous and metachronous cancers.

2. How common are bilateral synchronous breast cancers?

3. What histologic subtype of breast cancer has the highest likelihood of bilaterality?

4. After a unilateral diagnosis of breast cancer is made, what is the patient's risk of developing a contralateral cancer?

Bilateral Breast Cancer

1. Synchronous cancers refer to bilateral cancers that are detected simultaneously. Metachronous cancers are bilateral cancers not detected simultaneously but, rather, found at different points in time.

2. Approximately 5–10% of cancers are bilateral with MRI screening of the contralateral breasts.

3. Bilaterality is highest with invasive lobular carcinoma. The incidence is approximately 30% of cases.

4. Based on the literature (prior to contralateral MRI screening), the risk of developing metachronous cancer in the opposite breast is approximately 1% per year.

References

Lee SG, Orel SG, Woo IJ, Cruz-Jove E, Putt ME, Solin LJ, Czerniecki BJ, Schnall MD: MR imaging screening of the contralateral breast in patients with newly diagnosed breast cancer: Preliminary results, *Radiology* 226:773–778, 2003.

Murphy TJ, Conant EF, Hanau CA, Ehrlich SM, Feig SA: Bilateral breast carcinoma: Mammographic and histologic correlation, *Radiology* 195:617, 1995.

Cross-Reference

Ikeda, *Breast Imaging: THE REQUISITES*, p 214.

Comment

Bilateral breast carcinoma is uncommon and is usually divided into two subtypes, metachronous and synchronous lesions, based on the time of presentation of the cancers. Metachronous lesions are contralateral breast cancers that are diagnosed at different points in time, frequently many years apart. The exact incidence of metachronous carcinomas is difficult to determine because a cancer detected at a later time in the contralateral breast may actually be a metastasis from an already present breast carcinoma in the other breast.

Synchronous carcinomas refer to cancers that are detected bilaterally, at the same time. Synchronous cancers were once thought to be quite rare; however, the incidence is increasing with the use of MRI screening of the contralateral breast at the time of diagnosis of a unilateral breast cancer. Some series report a 5–10% incidence of bilaterality with contralateral breast screening in patients with known unilateral cancer (with the contralateral synchronous cancer being occult to routine mammographic imaging and breast exam).

There is a varying likelihood of bilaterality in breast cancers based on histologic subtypes; invasive lobular carcinoma has the highest incidence of bilaterality, with some reports of up to 30%. Invasive ductal carcinoma, although more frequent, has a lower reported incidence of bilaterality because many of the contralateral foci of metachronous cancer are thought to be metastases from the already diagnosed (and frequently treated) cancer in the other breast. In one series describing bilateral breast cancers, the cancers tended to have the same imaging appearance and be located in the same quadrants (mirror image and mirror locations) as in this case.

Overall, the risk of developing bilateral cancers is reported to be approximately 1% per year, which is approximately six times higher than that of the general population. Therefore, patients with a unilateral prior diagnosis of breast cancer are considered high risk in terms of screening the contralateral breast.

Notes

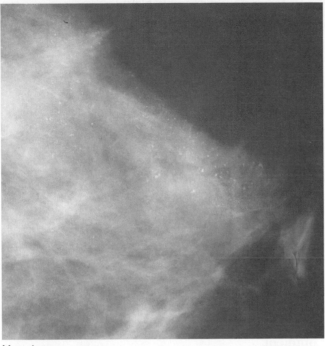

Mag view

1. The patient presents with the clinical symptoms of "nipple irritation and scaling." Based on the clinical findings, what diagnosis must be considered?

2. Describe the mammographic findings and give a BI-RADS category.

3. How common are mammographic findings in this clinical entity?

4. What is the clinical management of this process if malignant?

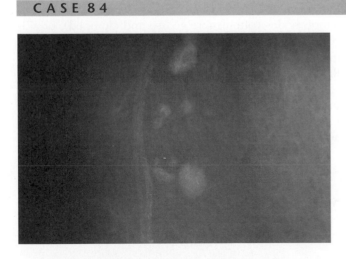

1. Is there anything unusual about the lymph nodes seen on the cropped mammogram image of the left axilla?

2. What is in your differential diagnosis?

3. What is the next step in the workup?

4. What is the BI-RADS category for this mammogram?

C A S E 8 3

Paget's Disease

1. Paget's disease of the nipple.

2. Mammographically, there are segmentally distributed pleomorphic calcifications extending from the nipple and subareolar area to the lateral breast.

3. Approximately 50% of the time there are associated suspicious mammographic findings when a patient presents with the clinical entity of Paget's disease of the nipple.

4. When the nipple is involved in malignancy, it is usually surgically removed.

Reference

Echevarria JJ, Lopez-Ruiz JA, Martin D, Imaz I, Martin M: Usefulness of MRI in detecting occult breast cancer associated with Paget's disease of the nipple–areolar complex, *Br J Radiol* 77:1036–1039, 2004.

Cross-Reference

Ikeda, *Breast Imaging: THE REQUISITES*, p 305.

Comment

Paget's disease of the nipple represents 1–5% of all breast cancers and is characterized by malignant ductal cells extending to the nipple surface through the terminal lactiferous ducts. Early clinical findings are limited to the nipple and may include reddening, scaling, or crusting of the nipple surface and associated puritis. There may also be areolar thickening and nipple retraction. Approximately 50% of the time, the mammogram will be normal, and to make the diagnosis of cancer a wedge biopsy of the abnormal nipple is necessary.

A thorough imaging workup is necessary since the disease may not be confined to just the nipple. Mammography may show ductal calcifications or a subareolar mass that was clinically unsuspected. Ultrasound is useful if there is a palpable mass or mammographically detected focal density that may be due to an invasive component of the disease. Because of the reported high incidences of multifocal and multicentric lesions in the breast, mastectomy with nodal dissection was frequently done in the past. However, with improved imaging staging, such as MR, selected cases may now have breast conservation.

Notes

C A S E 8 4

Gold Deposits in Lymph Nodes

1. The lymph nodes contain tiny bright, metal-density deposits.

2. The tiny foci could represent gold from therapy for rheumatoid arthritis. Granulomatous diseases can cause calcifications to develop in lymph nodes. Rarely, metastatic spread of breast cancer may be seen in a lymph node.

3. No further workup is needed in this case.

4. BI-RADS category 2: benign.

Reference

Bruwer A, Nelson GW, Spark RP: Punctate intranodal gold deposits simulating microcalcifications on mammograms, *Radiology* 163:87–88, 1987.

Cross-Reference

Ikeda, *Breast Imaging: THE REQUISITES*, p 304.

Comment

Tiny opacities are seen in all lymph nodes seen on this mammogram, including an intramammary node on the right and all axillary nodes. This is an unusual appearance, but it is most often due to a benign cause.

Rheumatoid arthritis can be treated with gold therapy, also termed chrysotherapy. The ingested gold can be transported to the nodes, which are then seen on the mammogram as metallic particles in the lymph nodes.

In the differential diagnosis, you can consider granulomatous disease, which can cause calcifications in lymph nodes (often more coarse and clumped), or silicone in lymph nodes if the patient has had silicone implants or injections, either present or in the past. Rarely, breast cancer that presents as microcalcification could cause axillary node calcifications, but this is unlikely to be so widespread. Also, in metastatic involvement, the lymph nodes would likely be enlarged and dense.

This patient has been on gold therapy for rheumatoid arthritis.

Notes

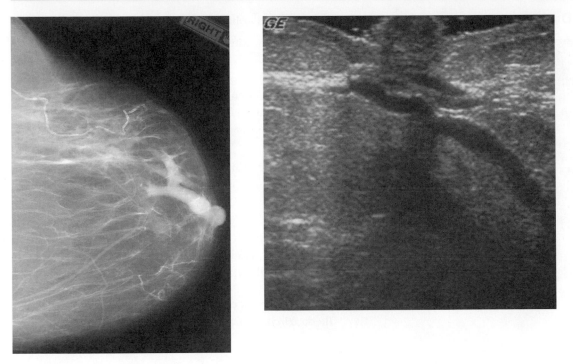

1. This is the baseline mammogram in a 55-year-old woman. Describe the mammographic findings.

2. What is the differential diagnosis?

3. What might be the next diagnostic test or clinical question?

4. What is the BI-RADS category?

Solitary Dilated Duct

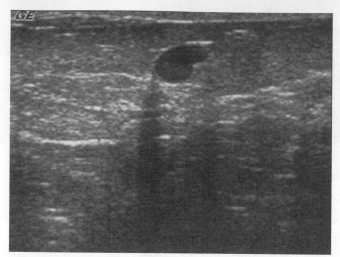

US of duct with dependent debris

1. There is a solitary dilated duct.

2. Papilloma, intraductal carcinoma, or benign duct ectasia.

3. Questioning and physical exam of the patient are needed to determine if there is nipple discharge. Additional imaging either with ultrasound or MRI could be considered to look for an intraductal lesion.

4. If no other clinical findings or imaging lesions, BI-RADS category 3: probably benign with short-term follow-up recommended.

Reference

Pisano ED, Braeuning MP, Burke E: Case 8: Solitary intraductal papilloma, *Radiology* 210:795, 1999.

Cross-Reference

Ikeda, *Breast Imaging: THE REQUISITES*, p 293.

Comment

The most important fact about a solitary dilated duct is whether it is new; careful comparison to old films is needed. If there are no old films to assure stability, an intraductal lesion causing the dilation must be searched for. The patient should be questioned about any history of nipple discharge. On ultrasound, the duct should be easily identified and should be evaluated for any intraductal lesions.

Benign papillomas are the most likely cause of ductal dilatation, and occasionally dystrophic calcifications may be seen mammographically. However, intraductal carcinomas may also cause ductal dilatation with or without suspicious calcifications. Biopsy may be necessary to determine the cause when calcifications are present or the duct is changing over time. Ultrasound or MRI may be helpful to define intraductal lesions; however, papillomas and small intraductal carcinomas may look similar. In the absence of a history of discharge or a definable lesion (mammographic calcifications, ultrasound, or MRI lesions), the patient could be followed at short intervals to establish stability of the solitary dilated duct. This is a case of benign ductal ectasia.

Notes

CC view

US

This 53-year-old woman presents with bloody nipple discharge.

1. Describe the mammographic finding on the CC view.

2. Describe the ultrasound findings.

3. What is the most likely diagnosis?

4. Is a biopsy needed? If so, what type is recommended?

Papilloma

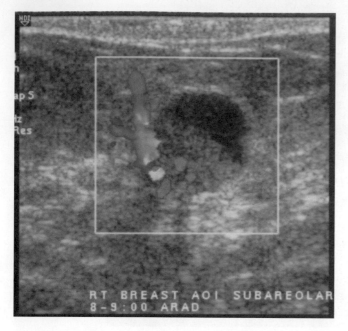

1. There is a mass with obscured margins just lateral to the nipple in the subareolar tissue.

2. The ultrasound demonstrates an intracystic mass that is highly vascular.

3. A solitary benign intracystic papilloma.

4. Yes, a biopsy is necessary to exclude malignancy. The choice of either an excisional or core biopsy is controversial. However, with the newer and larger gauge vacuum-assisted core devices, core biopsy may be sufficient if there is no atypia seen histologically.

References

Berg WA: Image-guided breast biopsy and management of high-risk lesions, *Radiol Clin North Am* 42(5): 935–946, 2004.

Renshaw AA, Derhagopian RP, Tizol-Blanco DM, Gould EW: Papillomas and atypical papillomas in breast core needle biopsy specimens: Risk of carcinoma in subsequent excision, *Am J Clin Pathol* 122(2): 217–221, 2004.

Cross-Reference

Ikeda, *Breast Imaging: THE REQUISITES*, pp 113–116.

Comment

In a review of women with spontaneous nipple discharge, the vast majority (61%) had benign intraductal papillomas; only 6% had carcinoma. However, if the patient presents with either a palpable lump or a mass on mammography associated with the discharge, the incidence of cancer increases significantly.

Solitary benign papillomas are the most common benign papillary lesions and the most common intraductal mass. Papillomas develop in the major ducts and lactiferous sinuses of the subareolar breast tissue. They occur most commonly in peri- and postmenopausal women and are associated with no increased risk for breast carcinoma. Most patients with solitary, large-duct papillomas present with nipple discharge. Bloody nipple discharge may occur if the papilloma twists on its fibrovascular stalk and ischemia and necrosis occur. Clinically, clear nipple discharge may also occur due to secretory changes produced by the papilloma.

Mammographically, papillomas are round, often well-circumscribed subareolar masses that may contain amorphous or heterogeneous calcifications; alternatively, papillomas may present solely as a cluster of calcifications without a mammographically evident mass. Ductography may be helpful to localize the papilloma within the discharging duct, but frequently MRI gives a more global picture and may reveal additional lesions in women with nipple discharge.

Solitary duct papillomas have a characteristic low-power microscopic appearance; they appear in a dilated duct as a friable mass with a central fibrovascular core. Ductal proliferation and atypia may be seen in association with the papilloma, and there may be sclerosis of the fibrovascular core. Sclerosing papillomas can have a highly complex pattern, and the spectrum of atypical duct hyperplasia and *in situ* carcinoma may arise in a papilloma. For these reasons, historically when a papilloma was suspected based on imaging or clinical findings, surgical excision was usually recommended. However, recently, with the use of larger gauge vacuum-assisted core needles, there has been good concordance of core results compared to excisional biopsy results. However, if on core biopsy there is any form of cellular atypia or complexity seen pathologically, an excision of the papilloma is recommended. This case represents a benign intraductal papilloma.

Notes

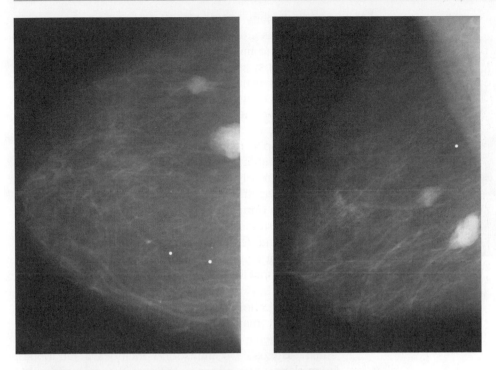

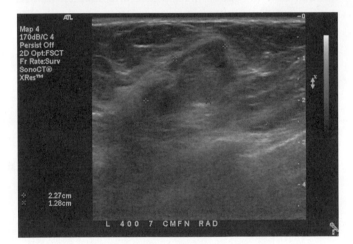

1. This patient is postmenopausal (age 58 years) and presents with increasing pain in the left breast. Is this a worrisome presentation?

2. Are the mammographic findings suspicious?

3. Is ultrasound useful in this patient? Why?

4. Are the masses suspicious on ultrasound?

Mucinous Cancer

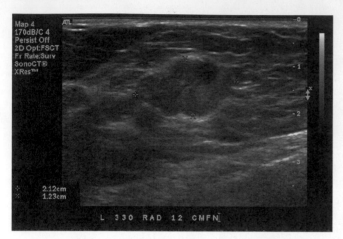

1. New-onset pain in the postmenopausal woman is concerning, particularly if the patient is not taking hormone replacement therapy.

2. There are two relatively dense masses in the left breast; further evaluation is needed, BI-RADS 0.

3. Yes, for further evaluation of the dense masses and to guide needle biopsy.

4. The masses are suspicious for malignancy because they are high density, with irregular shapes and microlobulated margins. The clinical presentation of new pain in a postmenopausal patient adds to the concern. Biopsy is indicated, and it was performed on both masses using ultrasound guidance.

References

Conant EF, Dillon RL, Palazzo J, Ehrlich SM, Feig SA: Imaging findings in mucin-containing carcinomas of the breast: Correlation with pathologic features, *Am J Roentgenol* 163:821–824, 1994.

Lam WWM, Chu WCW, Tse GM, Ma TK: Sonographic appearance of mucinous carcinoma of the breast, *Am J Roentgenol* 182(4):1069–1074, 2004.

Cross-Reference

Ikeda, *Breast Imaging: THE REQUISITES*, pp 106, 146.

Comment

Two masses were seen in the left breast in this patient with left breast pain. She had not had a mammogram performed for 5 years, and no prior films were available at the time of presentation. The mammogram demonstrates dense masses in the left posterior breast, easily seen in the fatty breast. In evaluating suspicious masses, ultrasound is a useful tool, particularly if you are going to proceed to image-guided needle biopsy. Ultrasound-guided biopsy is quicker to perform than stereotactic biopsy and usually easier for the patient to tolerate. Ultrasound imaging allows "real-time" imaging, which may improve the accuracy of biopsy.

The masses are relatively deep in the left lateral breast. Despite their size, they were difficult to detect on ultrasound imaging. This may due to the fact that the masses are nearly isoechoic to surrounding fat. In mucinous cancer, the classic presentation is a relatively dense mass on mammography and a mass isoechoic to fat on ultrasound.

Ultrasound features of the pure mucinous cancer are different from those of invasive ductal cancer, not otherwise specified. The mucinous cancer on ultrasound may have relatively benign features: well-defined with a thin echogenic capsule isoechoic to surrounding fat. Or they may have more suspicious features of a thick echogenic halo and irregular margins. The differential diagnosis on ultrasound includes a fat lobule, lipoma, and fibroadenomas. Since the masses in this patient are dense on mammogram, they are clearly not lipomas or fat lobules.

This patient's histopathology was pure mucinous carcinoma for both masses, low nuclear grade. The nodes were negative.

Notes

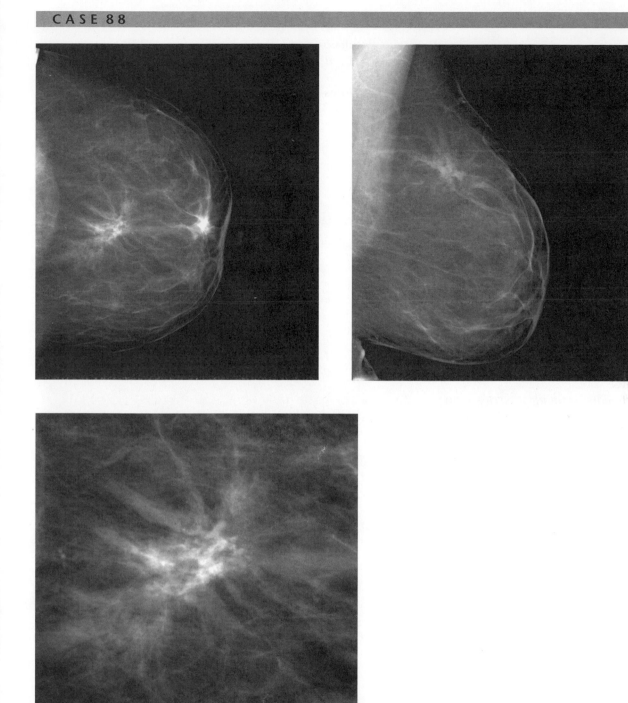

Mag view

1. This patient presented for her baseline screening study and a digital mammogram was performed. Describe the mammographic findings.

2. What is the most likely diagnosis and what BI-RADS category should be given?

3. What is the recommendation for the next procedure?

4. A core biopsy was performed and the results were "sclerosing adenosis." Is this concordant with the imaging finding?

Category 5 Lesion

1. There is large area of architectural distortion associated with a focal asymmetry in the upper breast. There are faint amorphous calcifications associated with the lesion.

2. The most likely diagnosis is an invasive ductal carcinoma, and a BI-RADS category 5: highly suspicious was given.

3. A core biopsy was recommended.

4. The lesion may actually be sclerosing adenosis or a radial scar, but the benign histologic results are discordant with the highly suspicious appearance. Excisional biopsy is necessary.

Reference

Gill HK, Ioffe OB, Berg WA: When is a diagnosis of sclerosing adenosis acceptable at core biopsy? *Radiology* 228:50–57, 2003.

Cross-Reference

Ikeda, *Breast Imaging: THE REQUISITES*, p 103.

Comment

This patient has a very remarkable baseline screening study. The digital mammogram shows a large area of focal asymmetry and architectural distortion in the upper right breast. The large spicules are associated with amorphous calcifications and extend anteriorly at least 8 cm toward the nipple. The immediate concern is that this lesion represents a large invasive ductal carcinoma. The patient was given a BI-RADS category 5: highly suspicious. A core biopsy was recommended. The likelihood of malignancy for a category 5 lesion is approximately 96%.

The results from the core biopsy were surprising: The pathologic diagnosis was sclerosing adenosis with no evidence of malignancy. Sclerosing adenosis is a lesion that arises from the lobule of the breast and is characterized histologically by the proliferation of acini. There may also be surrounding stromal proliferation, which compresses and elongates the acinar spaces and may cause architectural distortion mammographically or even a mass. Although sclerosing adenosis presents most frequently as a cluster of punctate, round, or amorphous calcifications, occasionally these lesions may present as palpable masses on breast exam.

In this case, the mammographic appearance is highly suspicious, and even though the biopsy results indicated sclerosing adenosis, the benign histologic findings and highly suspicious imaging findings are discordant. Malignancy must be excluded with excisional biopsy. On excision, the entire lesion was due to sclerosing adenosis and florid hyperplasia. There was no associated *in situ* or invasive carcinoma.

Notes

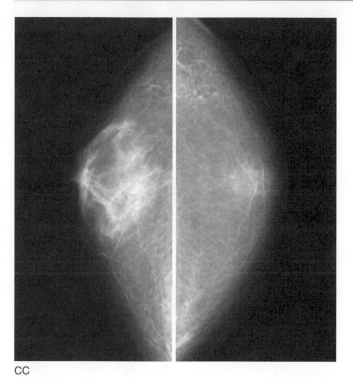

CC

1. What is the abnormality in this male patient who presents with a tender palpable left breast mass?
2. What is the typical age for this condition?
3. Is this condition rare?
4. What are the usual presenting symptoms?

Gynecomastia

1. Gynecomastia.

2. There are two peaks of increased incidence: in normal adolescents (high estradiol levels) and in older men with decreasing testosterone levels.

3. Common condition; 57% of men older than 44 years.

4. Tender, soft, palpable mass behind the nipple. Usually, gynecomastia is bilateral and asymmetric, but it may be unilateral. Rarely, it is bilaterally symmetric.

Reference

Appelbaum AH, Evans GFF, Levy KR, Amirkhan RH, Schumpert TD: Mammographic appearances of male breast disease, *RadioGraphics* 19:559–568, 1999.

Cross-Reference

Ikeda, *Breast Imaging: THE REQUISITES*, pp 279–280.

Comment

This patient is a 70-year-old male being treated for prostate cancer.

Gynecomastia is a common condition in men, and it is the most common reason for men to present for a mammogram. It is an overgrowth of ductal epithelium and stromal elements; it may be tender on exam and may be detected by the patient or the referring physician. The differential diagnosis for a palpable mass in a male includes breast cancer, lipoma, epithelial inclusion cyst, fat necrosis, lymph node, and hematoma.

Gynecomastia develops from high exogenous or endogenous estrogen levels or, in older men, a decrease in testosterone. Men who present with a mass should initially have a bilateral mammogram.

The mammogram in gynecomastia classically shows a fan-shaped area of density behind the nipple. The edges of the mass fade into the surrounding fat. There is a also nodular form in which the edges may be well circumscribed. The focal asymmetry seen can extend into the upper outer quadrant of the breast and is frequently asymmetric.

Ultrasound of the palpable finding may be important because gynecomastia can obscure a small cancer on the mammogram. On ultrasound, the entire area of gynecomastia should be evaluated for a hypoechoic mass. Cancer can coexist with gynecomastia and must be excluded.

Solid masses or complex cysts seen on ultrasound are suspicious for malignancy. Hyperechoic masses contiguous with the skin are typical for epidermal inclusion cysts. Fat necrosis has a varying appearance but is usually hyperechoic and may shadow. Lipomas are typically hyperechoic, located in the subdermal layer, oval in shape, and wider than tall. This is an example of asymmetric gynecomastia.

Notes

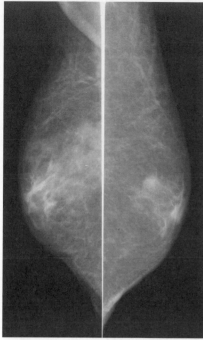
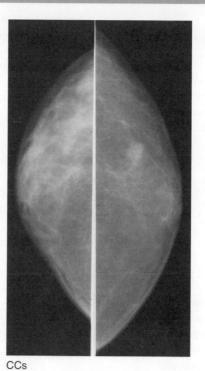

MLOs

CCs

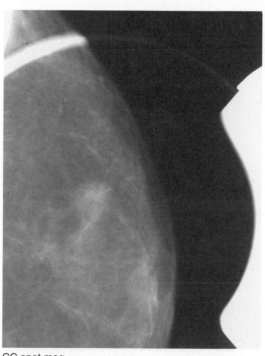

CC spot mag

1. This 60-year-old man presents with a palpable firm right breast lump. How should the workup begin?

2. Describe the mammographic findings.

3. What is the most likely diagnosis?

4. How common is breast cancer in males?

Male Breast Cancer

1. The workup should begin with a bilateral mammogram.

2. This patient has asymmetric gynecomastia (left greater than right). However, in the right lateral breast there is a poorly defined mass that on magnification views has heterogeneous calcifications.

3. Palpable masses in men may be benign lesions, such as lymph nodes or sebaceous cysts. However, this mass is very concerning because it is within the breast, is irregular, and has heterogeneous calcifications. This is most likely a primary breast cancer and a biopsy must be performed.

4. Male breast cancer accounts for less than 1% of all reported breast cancers and less than 0.2% of all cancers in men in the United States. Male breast cancer usually presents as a palpable mass that on mammography may be either a spiculated or a circumscribed mass and is often eccentrically located in the subareolar tissue or in the upper outer quadrant of the breast; calcifications are uncommon.

Reference

Appelbaum AH, Evans GFF, Levy KR, Amirkhan RH, Schumpert TD: Mammographic appearances of male breast disease, *RadioGraphics* 19:559–568, 1999.

Cross-Reference

Ikeda, *Breast Imaging: THE REQUISITES*, pp 279–280.

Comment

In evaluating men with breast lumps, a bilateral mammogram is the first study to perform because the lumps are most likely due to gynecomastia and benign breast tissue. A bilateral mammogram is helpful to compare for symmetry and to detected unsuspected gynecomastia in the contralateral breast for future follow-up. If the male is a teen or young adult, the workup may begin with a focused ultrasound since the incidence of cancer is extremely low. Ultrasound of the asymptomatic side may be helpful for comparison.

Typically, breast cancer in men presents as a firm painless mass in the subareolar region or slightly eccentric to the nipple. The overall prognosis for men with breast cancer is worse because men usually present at a later stage, when the mass is palpable. Nipple retraction or inversion or ulceration of the nipple are present in approximately 30% of cases, and bloody nipple discharge is common. Very few males who present with breast cancer are younger than 30 years old, but the incidence increases rapidly as age increases; in general,

younger men are more likely to have gynecomastia. The average age of men with breast cancer is slightly older than that of women (59 years vs late forties or early fifties for women). Risk factors for men to develop breast cancer include advanced age, exposure to ionizing radiation, cryptorchidism, testicular injury, Klinefelter syndrome, liver dysfunction, and family history of breast cancer.

Mammographically, breast cancer usually presents as a spiculated or well-defined mass. Calcifications are uncommon in male breast cancer; however, they are present in the case presented here. Gynecomastia usually presents in the subareolar area and shows a mottled density with fat, and on ultrasound it has an appearance of hypoechoic glandular tissue similar to the appearance of developing breast tissue in the pubescent female breast. Eccentric masses away from the subareolar location are suspicious for carcinoma.

Approximately 85% of male breast cancers are invasive ductal carcinomas. Biopsy such as a core biopsy performed under ultrasound guidance is necessary to confirm the diagnosis of malignancy.

Notes

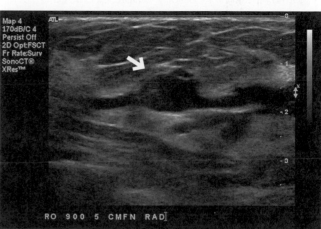

The BB locates the nipple in this patient who presents with a bloody nipple discharge.

1. What is the mammographic finding?

2. What is the ultrasound finding?

3. What should be done next?

4. What is the most common reason for bloody nipple discharge?

Intraductal Mass on Ultrasound

1. The mammogram shows ductal ectasia.

2. The ultrasound exam shows an intraductal mass.

3. The next step is to obtain histologic diagnosis.

4. Ninety percent of bloody nipple discharge is caused by benign papilloma.

References

Accuracy of core needle biopsy diagnosis in assessing papillary breast lesions: Histologic predictors of malignancy, *Mod Pathol*, 2003.

Mercado CL: Papillary lesions of the breast at percutaneous core-needle biopsy, *Radiology* 238:801–808, 2006.

Rosen EL: Imaging-guided core needle biopsy of papillary lesions of the breast, *Am J Roentgenol* 179:1185–1192, 2002.

Cross-Reference

Ikeda, *Breast Imaging: THE REQUISITES*, p 140.

Comment

Intraductal masses in the breast may be difficult to recognize mammographically but can be well seen on ultrasound, especially if, as in this case, the duct is focally dilated. The fluid in the duct provides the contrast needed to see the mass. Intraductal masses most commonly are due to papillary lesions, but they may also be seen in DCIS.

Papillary masses can develop in a duct or, less commonly, in a cyst. It is possible that what appears to be a cyst may in fact be a portion of a focally dilated duct. Papillary masses most commonly present as solitary masses in a large duct near the nipple. Multiple papillomas most commonly occur in smaller, more peripheral ducts.

Histologic diagnosis is needed to exclude intraductal cancer. Some experts advocate excisional biopsy, rather than core biopsy, when an intraductal mass is detected. Pathologists may not be able to differentiate benign from malignant papilloma by core biopsy alone. The relatively small volume of tissue obtained in a core biopsy may underestimate the severity of disease. However, with larger gauge, vacuum-assisted core biopsy, adequate material may be obtained to provide histologic diagnosis.

Recent reports suggest that papillary lesions diagnosed on core biopsy be surgically excised, as many may contain ADH or DCIS.

Notes

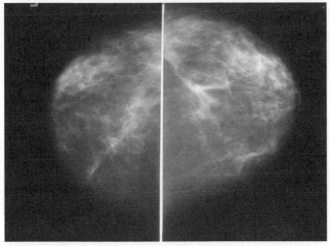

Initial CC views

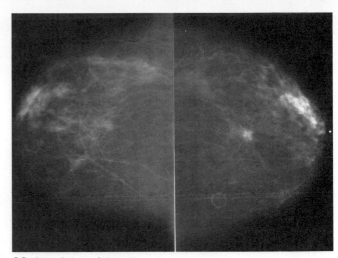

CC views 6 years later

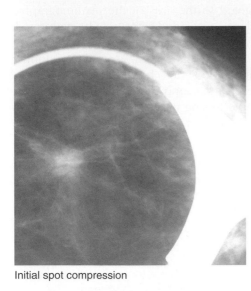

Initial spot compression

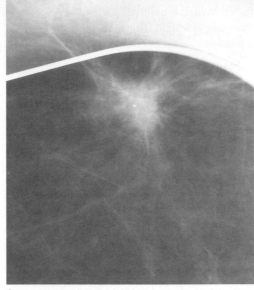

Spot compression 6 years later

1. What is the mammographic finding?

2. What is your differential diagnosis?

3. What is the appropriate management? BI-RADS category?

4. Compare the spot mammograms from the two exams. Does this change your management decision?

Architectural Distortion

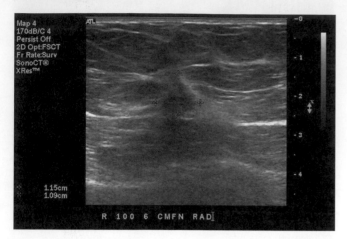

1. There is architectural distortion in the central right breast, changing only slightly over 6 years.

2. Differential diagnosis includes invasive cancer, radial scar, postsurgical changes, spiculated fat necrosis, and sclerosing adenosis.

3. Patient history should be obtained regarding surgical history. Because there is a possibility of malignancy, biopsy should be performed. BI-RADS 4.

4. The architectural distortion was followed for several years because of lack of interval change. However, stability of a suspicious finding should not change the management decision.

References

Rosen EL: Malignant lesions initially subjected to short term mammographic follow up, *Radiology* 223:221, 2002.

Varas X, Leborgne JH, Leborgne F, Mezzera J, Jaumandreu S, Leborgne F: Revisiting the mammographic follow-up of BI-RADS category 3 lesions, *Am J Roentgenol* 179:691–695, 2002.

Cross-Reference

Ikeda, *Breast Imaging: THE REQUISITES*, pp 28, 103.

Comment

There is a focus of architectural distortion in the right central breast, detected on a baseline mammogram, assigned to BI-RADS category 3, and followed. Subsequent mammograms failed to show any appreciable change to the eye of the reviewing radiologists. The architectural distortion was believed to be due to overlapping normal structures rather than a spiculated mass.

When assigning a mammographic finding to a follow-up (BI-RADS 3) or to biopsy (BI-RADS 4 or 5), the percentage chance of malignancy must be estimated. If the chance of malignancy is less than 2%, the lesion may be followed. Indeed, the likelihood of cancer developing in lesions initially assigned category 3 status is between 0.3 and 1.7% in published studies.

In reviewing mammograms, it is useful to compare prior films that are more than 6 months or 1 year old. Sometimes the finding changes so little during the 6-month or 1-year interval that it appears the same. If the same lesion is compared to an older film, a subtle change in size or density may be seen.

Ultrasound can be a useful adjunct tool in the setting of a mammographic finding that is indeterminate. Ultrasound targeted to the area of the mammographic lesion may disclose a mass, and biopsy can be performed. An area of mammographic architectural distortion that corresponds to a mass lesion on ultrasound is no longer "probably benign" and should be biopsied.

In this patient, ultrasound did demonstrate a mass, which was sampled using ultrasound-guided core technique. Low-grade infiltrating ductal carcinoma was the histologic diagnosis.

Notes

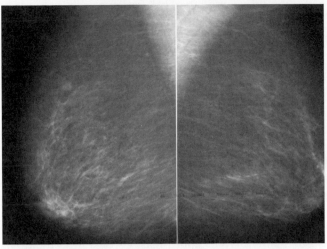

Initial MLO views

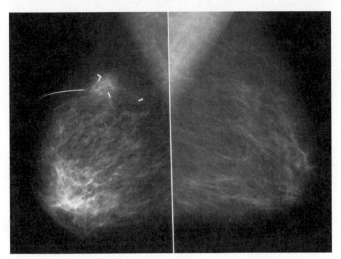

MLO views 1 year later

1. This patient has had lumpectomy and radiation therapy for breast cancer. Describe the findings.

2. What are the findings in the mammogram 1 year after diagnosis due to?

3. Are these changes expected?

4. How do recurrences usually present?

Breast Conservation Therapy

1. There is a small mass in the left upper outer breast in the initial mammogram. In the mammogram from one year later, there are changes compatible with breast conservation therapy.

2. There is skin thickening and thickening of the interstitial markings in the breast, consistent with edema. There is architectural distortion at the biopsy site, where there are surgical clips. There is a focal mass density at the biopsy site, consistent with hematoma/seroma.

3. These changes are expected after breast conservation therapy and will decrease over time.

4. A recurrence can appear as a mass, distortion, or calcifications. All of these findings can also be seen due to fat necrosis after breast conservation therapy.

References

Bloomer WD, Berenberg AL, Weissman BN: Mammography of the definitively irradiated breast, *Radiology* 118:425–428, 1976.

Brenner RJ, Pfaff JM: Mammographic features after conservation therapy for malignant breast disease: Serial findings standardized by regression analysis, *Am J Roentgenol* 167:171–178, 1996.

Liberman L, Van Zee KJ, Dershaw DD, Morris EA, Abramson AF, Samli B: Mammographic features of local recurrence in women who have undergone breast-conserving therapy for ductal carcinoma *in situ*, *Am J Roentgenol* 168:489–493, 1997.

Cross-Reference

Ikeda, *Breast Imaging: THE REQUISITES*, p 239.

Comment

Breast conservation therapy is the treatment of the breast for cancer that maintains the breast, as an alternative to mastectomy. Surgical excision of the tumor (lumpectomy) and radiation therapy to the whole breast, and sometimes to the chest wall and axilla, are performed. There are expected changes that are seen in the treated breast, including the following:

Increased interstitial markings throughout the breast and skin thickening due to edema
Architectural distortion at the lumpectomy site
Hematoma/seroma at the lumpectomy site
Calcifications may develop within the surgical bed and radiation field due to fat necrosis.

These findings may be seen in the first follow-up mammogram after radiation therapy is completed (usually 6 months after completion). All findings usually decrease in prominence over time, during the next 5 years, except for calcifications of fat necrosis, which commonly persist.

The follow-up interval for mammograms after breast conservation therapy is somewhat controversial. Some radiologists follow with mammograms of the affected side every 6 months for approximately 2 to 3 years, with annual mammograms of the nonaffected side. This approach is based on the fact that any recurrence or residual disease seen in the first few years will be detected early. The expected changes caused by the therapy can be recognized as they occur and then recede. In addition, the close follow-up after breast conservation therapy creates a new "baseline" to compare with future images. Others perform annual diagnostic mammograms after breast conservation therapy.

Newly developing, suspicious findings in the breast treated with conservation therapy may be related to residual disease, undetected at the time of initial treatment, or recurrence. Mammographic abnormalities seen in the first 2 years following treatment are believed to most likely represent residual disease, whereas those developing after 2 years may be recurrence. The recurrent disease may be seen at the site of treatment or may be in another quadrant of the breast. Residual and recurrent disease is typically seen at the lumpectomy site.

Hematomas that develop at the lumpectomy site need not be aspirated. They may be quite difficult to aspirate due to organization of the clot with fibrin. If they are symptomatic, painful, or inflamed, surgical drainage may be indicated.

Ultrasound of the lumpectomy site can be performed if there is concern that the developing mass at the site may be tumor rather than fluid collection. Hematoma may contain low-level internal echoes but should have no flow on Doppler interrogation.

Notes

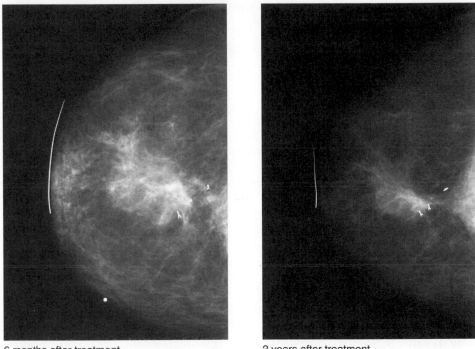

6 months after treatment   2 years after treatment

1. Describe the mammographic findings in the CC view of the left breast 6 months after treatment.

2. Describe the interval change in the breast between the two exams.

3. Why is the muscle tented?

4. Is biopsy indicated?

Breast Conservation Therapy

1. There is a focal asymmetry in the central adjacent to surgical clips, skin thickening, trabecular thickening, and architectural distortion, consistent with breast conservation therapy.

2. The asymmetry decreased in size, and skin thickening and increased trabecular thickening have decreased.

3. The muscle is a benign change due to the healing and retraction of the surgical bed. The retraction is accentuated by compression during mammography.

4. Biopsy is not indicated on the basis of the mammographic findings. If the patient has symptoms of increasing pain or lump, additional imaging should be performed with ultrasound, searching for recurrence not evident mammographically.

References

Brenner RJ, Pfaff JM: Mammographic features after conservation therapy for malignant breast disease: Serial findings standardized by regression analysis, *Am J Roentgenol* 167:171–178, 1996.

Dershaw DD, Shank B, Reisinger S: Mammographic findings after breast cancer treatment with local excision and definitive irradiation, *Radiology* 164:455–461, 1987.

Cross-Reference

Ikeda, *Breast Imaging: THE REQUISITES*, p 239.

Comment

After surgery and radiation, a hematoma or seroma is often seen at the lumpectomy site. Surgeons may place clips at the site to aid the radiation therapist in locating the site. The fluid-filled cavity is an expected finding but may make it difficult to evaluate for residual tumor or recurrent tumor at the site. Notice also the changes in breast irradiation in the initial film, which resolve by the second exam: skin thickening and trabecular prominence indicating breast and skin edema.

Ultrasound of the lumpectomy site should be performed if there is a clinically suspicious finding, such as increasing pain or palpable lump. A hematoma or seroma is a complex fluid structure filling the operative cavity. This fluid collection should decrease in size and become less dense over time, as in this case. Any increase in size should be treated with suspicion, and ultrasound should be performed to check for evidence of mass.

Notes

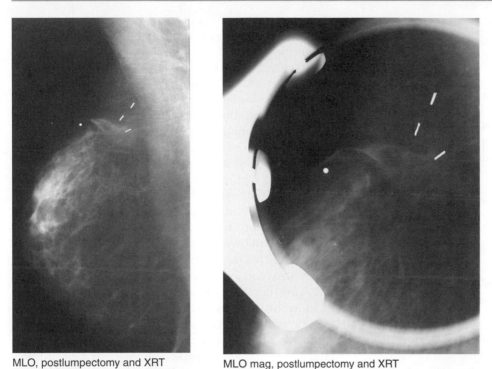

MLO, postlumpectomy and XRT

MLO mag, postlumpectomy and XRT

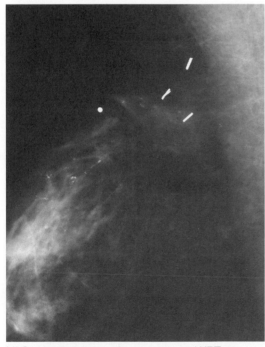

MLO mag, 3 years postlumpectomy and XRT

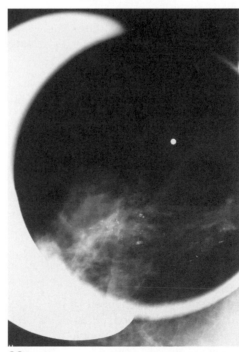

CC mag

1. This patient is status postlumpectomy and radiation therapy for invasive ductal carcinoma with an extensive *in situ* component. Magnification views of the surgical bed are shown from the 2-year and 3-year follow-up studies. Describe the findings in the 3-year follow-up magnification view.

2. Name risk factors for recurrence of cancer in patients who have undergone breast conservation therapy.

3. Is this case more likely a treatment failure or a new breast cancer arising in the same breast?

4. What is the treatment recommendation for this patient following these imaging findings?

Recurrence at Lumpectomy

1. There are pleomorphic calcifications in a linear distribution extending anteriorly from the site of prior surgery.

2. Risk factors include a young age at presentation (younger than 35 years), an invasive ductal carcinoma with an extensive intraductal component, a ductal carcinoma *in situ* larger than 2.5 cm, close or positive margins following surgery at the original presentation, and no or inadequate treatment of the surgical bed with radiation therapy.

3. This is most likely a case of residual or recurrent tumor at the margin of the surgical and radiation treatment bed. This would be considered a treatment failure.

4. This patient most likely will undergo mastectomy once the diagnosis of recurrence has been established by percutaneous core biopsy.

References

Giess CS, Keating DM, Osborne MP, Rosenblatt R: Local tumor recurrence following breast-conservation therapy: Correlation of histopathologic findings with detection method and mammographic findings, *Radiology* 212:829–835, 1999.

Giess CS, Keating DM, Osborne MP, Mester J, Rosenblatt R: Comparison of rate of development and rate of change for benign and malignant breast calcifications at the lumpectomy bed, *Am J Roentgenol* 175:789–793, 2000.

Cross-Reference

Ikeda, *Breast Imaging: THE REQUISITE*, p 246.

Comment

This patient presents with a treatment failure with mammographically detected suspicious calcifications extending from the margin of the surgical bed toward the nipple. Benign fat necrosis developing in the biopsy site may mimic recurrence, and this patient underwent a stereotactic core biopsy to establish the diagnosis of recurrent *in situ* comedo carcinoma. She then underwent mastectomy because she was no longer eligible for additional radiation therapy.

In patients with recurrence, the diagnosis is made mammographically in approximately 50% of patients and by physical exam in the other 50%. Mammographically detected recurrences are most commonly detected as suspicious calcifications or masses, but the mammographic appearance of the recurring tumor is frequently similar to the mammographic appearance of the original tumor. The palpable recurrences most often are invasive cancers. Recurrent or residual tumors in radiated breasts frequently arise along the margin of the lumpectomy bed. Tumors occurring distant to the primary site often have an appearance similar to the primary lesion and occur at the same rate as tumors in a contralateral breast. Tumors that arise distant to the treated bed are thought to represent new tumors rather than residual tumors or recurrent tumors.

Risk factors for treatment failure in breast conservation include young age at the time of presentation (<35 years) and patients who are treated for an invasive ductal carcinoma with an extensive intraductal component, as in this case. Of course, close or positive margins are a contraindication to breast conservation, and careful evaluation following lumpectomy for calcifications is necessary. This patient had no residual calcifications on her postexcision mammogram, which was performed following her lumpectomy and prior to the initiation of radiation therapy. Histologically, her margins were thought to be clear of tumor. She did, however, have an extensive intraductal component and her tumor was larger than 2.5 cm at presentation; such large tumors with an extensive intraductal component frequently have microscopic skip lesions extending along the ductal system toward the nipple.

Notes

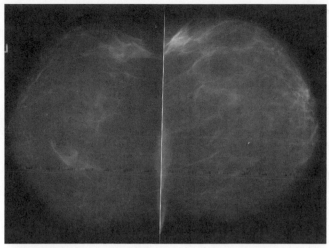

Initial CC

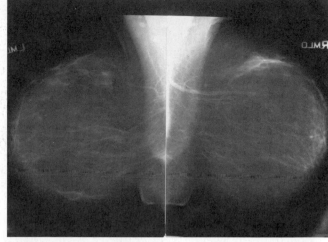

Initial MLO

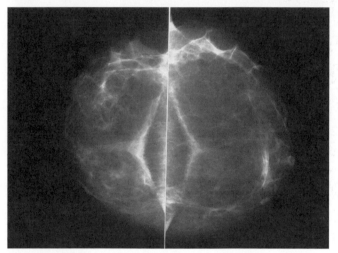

CC 2 years later

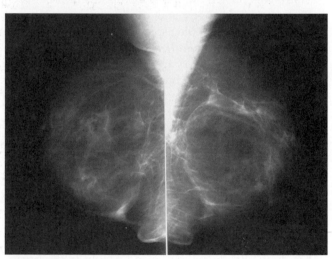

MLO 2 years later

1. What are the changes in this woman's mammogram over the 2 years?

2. What are the expected changes on the mammogram in this circumstance?

3. Is there an increased risk of breast cancer with this surgery?

4. Can subsequent cancer be difficult to find due to the surgical change?

Reduction Mammoplasty

1. There is a change in the size of the breast, and there are typical scar lines and shift of breast tissue seen with reduction mammoplasty.

2. Architectural distortion, calcifications, and fat lucency.

3. No.

4. Yes, scarring can mimic the architectural distortion of malignancy.

References

Brinton LA, Persson I, Boice JD Jr, McLaughlin JK, Fraumeni JF Jr: Breast cancer risk in relation to amount of tissue removed during breast reduction operations in Sweden, *Cancer* 91(3):478–483, 2001.

Mitnick JS, Vazquez MF, Plesser KP, Pressman PI, Harris MN, Colen SR, Roses DF: Distinction between postsurgical changes and carcinoma by means of stereotaxic fine-needle aspiration biopsy after reduction mammaplasty, *Radiology* 188:457–462, 1993.

Tarone RE, Lipworth L, Young VL, McLaughlin JK: Breast reduction surgery and breast cancer risk: Does reduction mammaplasty have a role in primary prevention strategies for women at high risk of breast cancer? *Plast Reconstr Surg* 113(7):2104–2110, 2004.

Cross-Reference

Ikeda, *Breast Imaging: THE REQUISITES*, p 27.

Comment

Reduction mammoplasty is a relatively frequent surgery performed on the breast for cosmetic reasons. Usually, this is done to reduce the size and weight of the breast, but it may also be performed to "lift" the breast. The surgeon makes incisions in the breast, removes breast tissue, and then replaces the nipple higher on the mound of the breast. The incisions most commonly used are circumareolar, a vertical scar from the nipple to the inframammary fold, and a transverse incision along the inframammary fold.

The incisions made in the breast will lead to scar formation and not infrequently to fat necrosis. The scar tissue may develop calcifications. The most common mammography findings after reduction surgery are architectural distortion, punctuate calcifications, focal fat lucency, and lines of density along the scars, as seen in this case. Also, skin thickening is seen in the lower breast, at the scar, and the ducts may appear to terminate lower than the nipple location because the nipple has been moved up.

Technologists should always chronicle any breast surgery on the patient history form prior to performing the mammogram.

Patients may present with a palpable lump after reduction mammoplasty, often along the scar tissue. Mammographic views of the palpable finding should be performed, and if fat necrosis is seen, no further workup is necessary. The patient may want to be seen by her plastic surgeon for reassurance. If the mammogram shows no signs of fat necrosis, ultrasound of the palpable finding should be performed. Fat necrosis on ultrasound may have the appearance of a hypoechoic round mass with a thick echogenic border.

Notes

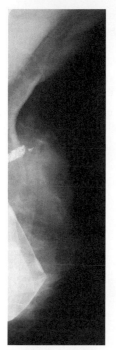
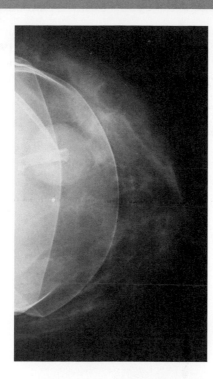

Patient A

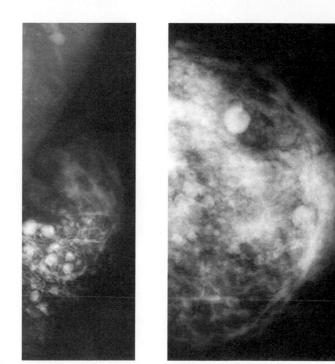

Patient B

1. Patient A complains of a decrease in the volume of the right breast. Why might this be?

2. What type of implant does patient A have?

3. Patient B complains of multiple lumps in the right breast. What procedure has this patient had?

4. What additional imaging would you recommend for the evaluation of the lumps?

Varieties of Augmentation

1. The implant has ruptured, causing a decrease in breast size.

2. A saline implant.

3. Injection of free silicone for augmentation.

4. Ultrasound to evaluate the areas of palpable concern; however, the free silicone will show areas of shadowing and the evaluation will be limited. MRI may also be helpful.

Reference

Caskey CI, Berg WA, Hamper UM, Sheth S, Chang BW, Anderson ND: Imaging spectrum of extracapsular silicone: Correlation of US, MR imaging, mammographic, and histopathologic findings, *RadioGraphics* 19:39–51, 1999.

Cross-Reference

Ikeda, *Breast Imaging: THE REQUISITES*, pp 252–270.

Comment

Patient A has saline implants. The elastomer, or shell of the implant, is made of silicone, but internal saline filling of the implant is more lucent than the silicone of the elastomer. The valve through which the saline is injected to fill the implant is also visible. Silicone implants are very dense because the optical density of silicone is higher than that of water or glandular tissue (oil implants are also low density). When saline implants rupture, the released saline is absorbed into the surrounding tissues and is usually not visible mammographically. This is in contrast to the high-density silicone that may be seen in extracapsular ruptures of silicone implants. The high-density tenacious material may be seen beyond the implant margin and may have visibly migrated into the breast tissue and axilla. When saline implants rupture, the wrinkled elastomer is often able to be felt by the patient.

Patient B has had injections of free silicone in the inferior aspect of the right breast. Many of the high-density nodules have rimlike calcifications due to the granulomatous response they have generated. Mammographic evaluation is quite difficult in these patients due to the high-density masses that may obscure areas of breast tissue. However, any area of spiculation or suspicious calcifications should prompt a recommendation for a biopsy. Ultrasound is also quite difficult to interpret in these patient due to the silicone granulomas and their associated intense shadowing. MRI may be helpful in evaluating areas of concern on breast exam or if there are equivocal findings on mammography. Injections of liquid silicone directly into the breast parenchyma were popular in the 1950s and 1960s but were banned in the 1970s due to adverse effects, including infection, fibrosis, lymphadenopathy, and the formation of silicone granulomata, which made physical exam and mammographic screening difficult.

Notes

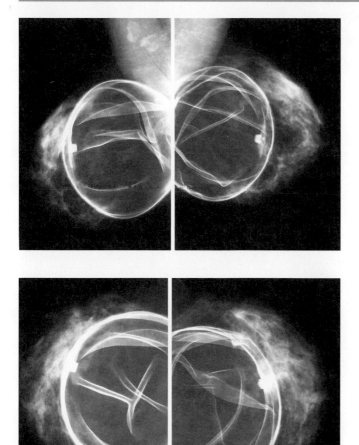

1. This patient has implants. What are the common materials used to fill the implants?

2. Can you tell if the implants are in front of or deep to the pectoral muscle?

3. Can you tell what material is in these implants?

4. Why is this type of implant no longer used?

Peanut Oil Implants

1. The most common materials are silicone and saline. Peanut oil was also used for a limited time.

2. These implants are in front of the pectoral.

3. These implants are filled with oil.

4. There was a high complication rate with oil implants.

References

Rizkalla M, Duncan C, Matthews RN: Trilucent breast implants: A 3 year series, *Br J Plast Surg* 54(2):125–127, 2001.

Young VL, Diehl GJ, Eichling J, Monsees BS, Destouet J: The relative radiolucencies of breast implant filler materials, *Plast Reconstr Surg* 91(6):1066–1072, 1993.

Young VL, Lund H, Ueda K, Pidgeon L, Schorr MW, Kreeger J: Bleed of and biologic response to triglyceride filler used in radiolucent breast implants, *Plast Reconstr Surg* 97(6):1179–1193, 1996.

Cross-Reference

Ikeda, *Breast Imaging: THE REQUISITES*, p 252.

Comment

Implants filled with peanut oil (triglycerides) were studied in the mid-1990s to improve the ability to see through the implant on mammography. The density of silicone is such that the breast parenchyma cannot be seen through the implant, and mammography is limited in these patients. Peanut oil is lucent, and studies on breast models showed that parenchyma could be visualized through the implant. Studies also showed that the implants were safe; that is, if the oil leaked, this was not dangerous to health, and the oil in the implant was not likely to become infected.

Later experience with the oil implants showed a 10% risk of deflation and an overall reoperation rate of 20% with the oil implants in one study. This high complication rate led to the voluntary recall of the triglyceride implant in 1999. They are rarely seen in routine breast imaging, compared to silicone and saline implants.

Implants can be placed behind or in front of the pectoral muscle. The location of the implant relative to the muscle should be mentioned in the mammogram report. There is a benefit to placement of the implant behind the pectoral muscle because more of the breast tissue can be imaged on the mammogram with the subpectoral location.

Notes

1. These two T2-weighted MRIs were performed on two different patients for evaluation of silicone implant integrity. Are the implants intact in each patient?

2. Describe the implant findings.

3. Is this intracapsular or extracapsular rupture?

4. Is it important to distinguish between intracapsular and extracapsular rupture?

Implant Leak on MRI

1. Both implants in these two different patients are ruptured.

2. The implant shell is displaced inward, and silicone is seen on both sides of the shell, indicating silicone outside the envelope.

3. This is intracapsular rupture. The silicone leak is contained inside the fibrous capsule.

4. Yes. Extracapsular rupture is silicone which is free in the breast, where it can cause silicone granulomas and can be associated with pain and palpable lump. Intracapsular rupture may be asymptomatic. Treatment (explantation) is more common with extracapsular leak.

References

Berg WA, Caskey CI, Hamper UM, Kuhlman JE, Anderson ND, Chang BW, Sheth S, Zerhouni EA: Single- and double-lumen silicone breast implant integrity: Prospective evaluation of MR and US criteria, *Radiology* 197:45–52, 1995.

Berg WA, Nguyen TK, Middleton MS, Soo MS, Pennello G, Brown SL: MR imaging of extracapsular silicone from breast implants: Diagnostic pitfalls, *Am J Roentgenol* 178(2):465–472, 2002.

Cross-Reference

Ikeda, *Breast Imaging: THE REQUISITES*, p 255.

Comment

MRI is a useful exam for evaluation of the silicone implant. It is more accurate than the mammogram and ultrasound exam of the implant, especially for intracapsular rupture. Sequences for silicone implant evaluation can include scout image in T1 weighted, axial T2 weighted, axial inversion recovery, and sagittal T2 weighted. Silicone is hyperdense on IR and hypodense on T2. The polymer shell is well seen on T2, as shown here.

There is no indication for evaluating *saline* implants with MRI. If saline implants rupture, they collapse, which should be obvious on clinical exam. The saline is readily absorbed.

In a population-based study of unreferred women with silicone implants (the study did not distinguish between those with or without symptoms), it was found that 55% had rupture of the implant on MRI. Of those with rupture, most were intracapsular; 22% were extracapsular.

On MRI, the implant shell is a discrete thin membrane. Any silicone seen on the outer side of this membrane constitutes a leak. The small amount of silicone gel seen on the surface of the shell creates the "subcapsular line" sign. Infolding of the shell, or "radial folds," can be normal.

However, if silicone is seen on both sides of the shell in an infolding loop, as in this example, this is a sign of rupture. This sign is termed the *noose* or *keyhole* sign.

A more dramatic example is the second case, in which the implant silicone polymer shell is seen collapsed inside the fibrous capsule. This is called the "linguini" sign.

The distinction between intracapsular and extracapsular leak can be important. With extracapsular leak, free silicone is seen in the breast or extending into the axilla. Free silicone may give rise to the formation of siliconomas or silicone granulomas. In an intracapsular leak, which is more common, the fibrous capsule or scar that forms around the implant contains the leak so that no free silicone or silicone granuloma are seen in the surrounding breast tissue.

Notes

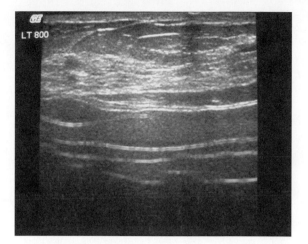

1. What does the ultrasound show in this asymptomatic patient with silicone implants?

2. What is the term for this ultrasound finding?

3. What does this sign correspond to on MRI?

4. Is ultrasound a reliable method for diagnosing implant rupture?

Intracapsular Rupture on Ultrasound

1. An intracapsular rupture of the silicone implant is seen, with horizontal echogenic lines within the implant envelope.

2. This is called the "stepladder" sign.

3. This corresponds to the "linguini" sign on MRI.

4. Ultrasound is useful in the diagnosis of implant rupture, although it is more sensitive for extracapsular rupture than intracapsular rupture.

References

Berg WA, Caskey CI, Hamper UM, Anderson ND, Chang BW, Sheth S, Zerhouni EA, Kuhlman JE: Diagnosing breast implant rupture with MR imaging, US, and mammography, *RadioGraphics* 13:1323–1336, 1993.

Chung KC, Wilkins EG, Beil RJ Jr, et al.: Diagnosis of silicone gel breast implant rupture by ultrasonography, *Plast Reconstr Surg* 97:104–109, 1996.

Cross-Reference

Ikeda, *Breast Imaging: THE REQUISITES*, p 262.

Comment

Ultrasound is useful for the evaluation of the integrity of silicone implants. Intracapsular rupture is a condition in which the silicone envelope collapses, but the silicone gel is contained within the fibrous capsule. The fibrous capsule is a scarlike shell that forms around the implant capsule after the surgery.

In intracapsular rupture the patient is often asymptomatic. In the stepladder sign, multiple horizontal linear echoes are seen which do not reach the lateral edge of the implant capsule. This represents the collapsed silicone envelope floating in the silicone gel.

Ultrasound is useful for evaluation of possible implant rupture because it is readily available and relatively inexpensive. It is more accurate for the diagnosis of implant rupture than mammography but not as accurate as MRI. If the classic findings of intracapsular or extracapsular rupture are seen on ultrasound, no further workup is needed. If there is strong clinical suspicious of implant rupture and ultrasound is negative, MRI may be indicated.

Notes

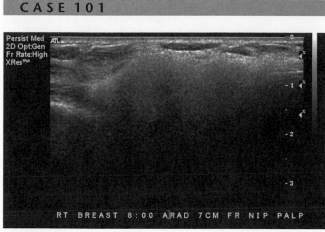

RT BREAST 8:00 ARAD 7CM FR NIP PALP

Palpable lump

1. This patient with silicone implants presents with a palpable lump. What is your differential diagnosis?

2. Based on the ultrasound image of the palpable lump, what is your diagnosis?

3. Is there need for another imaging study to confirm the diagnosis?

4. Is biopsy indicated?

Extracapsular Rupture on Ultrasound

1. The palpable lump may be due to breast mass or cyst, or may be silicone that has leaked from the implant.

2. The ultrasound appearance is characteristic of an extracapsular leak of silicone beyond the fibrous capsule into the adjacent breast tissue.

3. MRI can be performed but is not necessary if this ultrasound finding is seen.

4. No. The echogenic mass or "snowstorm" appearance finding represents free silicone in breast tissue. This is not a mass needing biopsy.

References

Caskey CI, Berg WA, Anderson ND, Sheth S, Chang BW, Hamper UM: Breast implant rupture: Diagnosis with US, *Radiology* 190:819–823, 1994.

Caskey CI, Berg WA, Hamper UM, Sheth S, Chang BW, Anderson ND: Imaging spectrum of extracapsular silicone: Correlation of US, MR imaging, mammographic, and histopathologic findings, *RadioGraphics* 19(90001):39–51, 1999.

Harris KM, Ganott MA, Shestak KC, Losken HW, Tobon H: Silicone implant rupture: Detection with US, *Radiology* 187:761–768, 1993.

Rosculet KA, Ikeda DM, Forrest ME, Oneal RM, Rubin JM, Jeffries DO, Helvie MA: Ruptured gel-filled silicone breast implants: Sonographic findings in 19 cases, *Am J Roentgenol* 159:711–716, 1992.

Cross-Reference

Ikeda, *Breast Imaging: THE REQUISITES*, p 262.

Comment

Extracapsular rupture of silicone implants may lead to a palpable lump, pain, and decrease in size of the implant. In evaluating the patient with silicone implants and a lump, a mammogram is the first imaging exam to perform. If the mammogram is normal, ultrasound is the next imaging study to perform. When scanning the palpable area, evaluate for a breast mass or cyst. Also check for extracapsular silicone. Leakage of silicone outside the confines of the implant envelope and the fibrous capsule causes a characteristic appearance on ultrasound. Free silicone is very hyperechoic with shadowing, which obscures posterior structures. This is termed the *snowstorm* appearance. The silicone may also be walled off by foreign body reaction and may calcify, forming a silicone granuloma, or "siliconoma." These granulomas are hypoechoic on ultrasound, and, if calcified, will shadow. Both the snowstorm and a granuloma are seen in this patient.

Rupture of silicone implants may be difficult to recognize mammographically. Look for a contour abnormality of the implant, which may represent a bulge in an intact implant or extravasated silicone. Silicone may be seen in axillary lymph nodes, but this is not absolutely diagnostic of rupture. It can also be seen when the patient has had a previous implant rupture and the old implant replaced.

If rupture is suspected based on the mammogram or because of clinical symptoms of pain, palpable mass, or softening of the implant, the next study can be ultrasound because it is less expensive and more readily available compared to MRI.

Notes

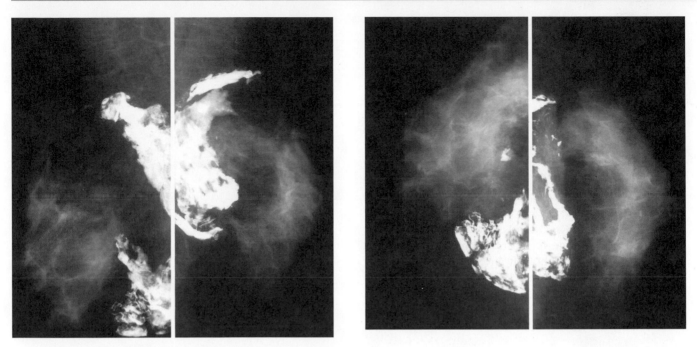

1. Describe the mammographic findings in this asymptomatic woman.

2. What is in your differential diagnosis?

3. Where are the calcifications anatomically?

4. Is surgery recommended?

Explanted Silicone Implants

1. Dense, plaque-like calcifications are seen in the posterior breast bilaterally.

2. This appearance is pathognomonic for removed silicone implants.

3. The calcifications are in the fibrous capsule, which had formed around the implant and was not removed when the implants were removed.

4. Surgery is not indicated.

References

Sinclair DS, Spigos DG, Olsen J: Case 2: Retained silicone and fibrous capsule in the right breast and retained fibrous capsule in the left breast after removal of implants, *Am J Roentgenol* 175(3):862–864, 2000.

Stewart NR, Monsees BS, Destouet JM, Rudloff MA: Mammographic appearance following implant removal, *Radiology* 185:83–85, 1992.

Cross-Reference

Ikeda, *Breast Imaging: THE REQUISITES*, p 262.

Comment

It is important to recognize the manifestations of silicone implant complications because they are frequently seen, and patients may present with pain or palpable findings that necessitate evaluation. Mammography, although intended for evaluation of possible breast cancer, is also a cost-effective, useful tool in evaluating the breast for residual silicone.

The fibrous capsule or the silicone envelope may be retained after explantation surgery. The capsule may have calcified prior to implant removal or may calcify later. Look for the spherical or collapsed shape of the calcified capsule in the expected location behind the glandular tissue, anterior to the pectoral muscle.

Silicone may migrate to the chest wall and axillary nodes and even to distant sites. This patient's breast may also include free silicone, which is difficult to differentiate from the dense calcification. The calcifications and dense fibrous capsule may mask developing breast masses and microcalcifications. Careful evaluation of these complicated mammograms is necessary to exclude malignancy.

Notes

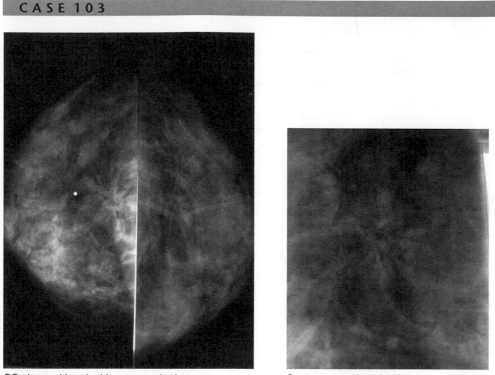

CC views with palpable area marked   Spot compression view

1. This is the patient's first mammogram. She presents with a palpable mass in her left breast. Describe the mammographic abnormality.

2. Can this lesion be determined to be benign or malignant on mammography?

3. What is the differential diagnosis?

4. How is the definitive diagnosis made?

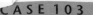

Radial Scar

1. There is a spiculated mass which corresponds to the palpable finding, with long, thin, radiating spicules against a background of fat. There is no central solid mass. Microcalcifications are present.

2. No, the pattern of architectural distortion with radiating spicules can be seen in malignancy and in benign radial scar.

3. The differential diagnosis is radial scar, invasive malignancy, and surgical scar.

4. The classic management was for excisional biopsy only because core needle biopsy may underestimate the disease. Radial scar may be associated with ADH, DCIS, and lobular neoplasia.

References

Adler DD, Helvie MA, Oberman HA, Ikeda DM, Bhan AO: Radial sclerosing lesion of the breast: Mammographic features, *Radiology* 176:737–740, 1990.

Brenner RJ, Jackman RJ, Parker SH, Evans WP III, Philpotts L, Deutch BM, Lechner MC, Lehrer D, Sylvan P, Hunt R, Adler SJ, Forcier N: Percutaneous core needle biopsy of radial scars of the breast: When is excision necessary? *Am J Roentgenol* 179(5):1179–1184, 2002.

Orel SG, Evers K, Yeh I, Troupin RH: Radial scar with microcalcifications: Radiologic–pathologic correlation, *Radiology* 183:479–482, 1992.

Cross-Reference

Ikeda, *Breast Imaging: THE REQUISITES*, p 103.

Comment

Radial scar is a pathologic abnormality consisting of a central sclerotic core radiating bands of proliferating ducts and lobules, which may entrap surrounding fat. Atypical cells may be within the benign stromal cells. The radiating bands of stromal cells cause a spiculated appearance on x-ray mammogram, which has an appearance similar to invasive cancer. Often in a radial scar, the spicules are thinner and longer than typically seen in malignancy, and there may be no central mass. The radiating spicules do not arise from a dense mass but, rather, converge in a central point that may have fat lucency, thus the term *dark star*.

When a mass is seen that could be a radial scar or an invasive cancer, pathology must be obtained. Traditionally, only an excisional biopsy was recommended because of the high association of the radial scar with DCIS, ADH, and ALH. It was believed that a small sample of the finding, such as is obtained with a core biopsy, may miss the associated finding. In addition, if the area is not well sampled, a radial scar can be confused with a tubular carcinoma by the pathologist.

However, since the mammographic abnormality may be an invasive cancer, and there is a benefit to performing the needle core biopsy in advance of excisional surgery, needle core biopsy can be performed as long as the lesion is excised if it is invasive cancer or a radial scar. If core biopsy is performed, a large-gauge needle (e.g., 10 or 11 gauge), particularly with vacuum assistance, will sample a larger proportion of the lesion. Multiple cores should be taken to increase the diagnostic yield of the biopsy. Knowledge of whether the lesion is invasive cancer or a radial scar is helpful prior to the definitive surgery so that the type of surgery can be planned and sentinel node biopsy can be performed if the lesion is malignant.

Notes

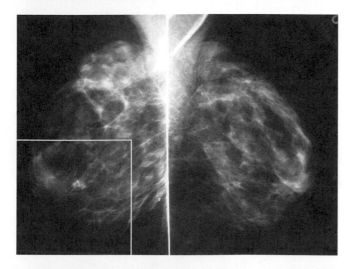

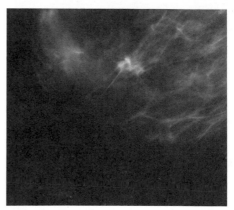

Left breast mag view

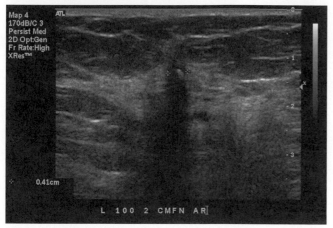

US of palpable area

1. This patient presents with a palpable mass in the left breast. Mammogram shows a focal density in the left central breast. What is the next step?

2. Describe the ultrasound findings.

3. Is biopsy indicated? BI-RADS?

4. If the tissue diagnosis is "stromal fibrosis" or "focal fibrosis," is this concordant with the imaging? How can you be sure you have biopsied the lesion?

Stromal Fibrosis

1. Ultrasound should be performed and correlated with the patient's palpable concern.

2. There is a hypoechoic area with posterior shadowing, which corresponds to the area of palpable concern.

3. A core biopsy should be performed. BI-RADS 4.

4. It may be concordant. Benign stromal or focal fibrosis can have an appearance that overlaps with malignant features on ultrasound and mammogram. A clip should be placed at the time of ultrasound-guided biopsy and a postbiopsy mammogram obtained. The location of the clip on the mammogram will confirm that the mammographic and ultrasound lesions are the same.

References

Harvey SC, Denison CM, Lester SC, DiPiro PJ, Smith DN, Meyer JE: Fibrous nodules found at large-core needle biopsy of the breast: Imaging features, *Radiology* 211:535–540, 1999.

Rosen EL, Soo MS, Bentley RC: Focal fibrosis: A common breast lesion diagnosed at imaging-guided core biopsy, *Am J Roentgenol* 173(6):1657–1662, 1999.

Sklair-Levy M, Samuels TH, Catzavelos C, Hamilton P, Shumak R: Stromal fibrosis of the breast, *Am J Roentgenol* 177(3):573–577, 2001.

Cross-Reference

Ikeda, *Breast Imaging: THE REQUISITES*, p 225.

Comment

Focal fibrosis or stromal fibrosis is a pathologic entity in which dense fibrosis occupies more than 90% of the interlobular stroma. This fibrous area may appear as an irregular mass on mammography and as a hypoechoic, irregular mass with dense shadowing on ultrasound. The finding may present clinically as a palpable mass.

When these imaging and clinical features are seen, biopsy needs to be performed to exclude malignancy. One of the responsibilities of performing needle core biopsy is to ensure that the imaging findings and the pathologic diagnosis are concordant—that is, that the pathologic diagnosis fits with your prebiopsy diagnosis. When imaging features that mimic malignancy are seen and the pathology is benign, reviewing the imaging findings is important.

In a published study, repeat biopsy was performed when fibrosis was diagnosed at pathology. The repeat biopsy confirmed the initial diagnosis. If you are certain that you sampled the lesion adequately, and the biopsy results are stromal fibrosis, follow-up imaging in 6 months should be recommended. If the mass increases in size or becomes more suspicious in appearance, repeat biopsy should be done to ensure malignancy is not present.

Notes

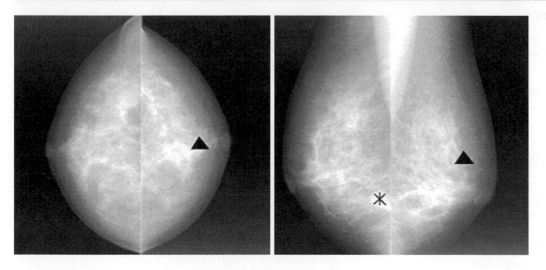

1. This is a mammogram after computer-aided detection (CAD) has been implemented. What do the overlying marks indicate?

2. When are the CAD images reviewed?

3. When the CAD system marks an abnormality, is it always cancer?

4. Can the system mark an area that is not a mass or calcifications?

Computer-Aided Detection

1. The triangles and asterisks are placed by the software to indicate areas of calcifications and mass.

2. Ideally, the CAD image is viewed following the review of the original mammogram. After CAD is seen, then take a second look at the mammogram to determine if the marks overlie true findings.

3. No. The system marks calcifications and densities that may be benign or malignant.

4. Yes. In an attempt to find subtle architectural distortion, the system will mark areas that are normal overlapping structures. CAD systems are very sensitive for microcalcifications but do not differentiate between benign and malignant.

References

Birdwell RL, Ikeda DM, O'Shaughnessy KF, Sickles EA: Mammographic characteristics of 115 missed cancers later detected with screening mammography and the potential utility of computer-aided detection, *Radiology* 219:192–202, 2001.

Destounis SV, DiNitto P, Logan-Young W, Bonaccio E, Zuley ML, Willison KM: Can computer-aided detection with double reading of screening mammograms help decrease the false-negative rate? Initial experience, *Radiology* 232:578–584, 2004.

Freer TW, Ulissey MJ: Screening mammography with computer-aided detection: Prospective study of 12,860 patients in a community breast center, *Radiology* 220:781–786, 2001.

Malich A, Sauner D, Marx C, Facius M, Boehm T, Pfleiderer SO, Fleck M, Kaiser WA: Influence of breast lesion size and histologic findings on tumor detection rate of a computer-aided detection system, *Radiology* 228:851–856, 2003.

Cross-Reference

Ikeda, *Breast Imaging: THE REQUISITES*, p 18.

Comment

CAD is used to attempt to increase the sensitivity of mammography. The rate of false-negative reading of mammography is reported to be as high as 25%. Some of these cancers are missed at screening because the malignancy cannot be detected on the mammogram, for instance, in the dense breast—so-called occult cancers. Others, however, may be missed because of the radiologist's failure to detect the abnormality which may be seen in hindsight. CAD is an effort to decrease false-negative mammograms by double reading the images.

Perception plays a major role in the optimization of mammography. Overcoming perceptual obstacles can allow the achievement of higher detection rates.

CAD is a system that checks the digital mammographic image for the presence of microcalcifications, masses, and distortion. It is used as a second reader. Once your initial interpretation has been done, a second look is taken at the CAD images to ensure that you did not overlook calcifications, a mass, or distortion. The system will place a designating symbol over an imaging finding that may be significant. The CAD image has many "false" marks, such as marking overlapping lines as spiculation. CAD is more accurate for calcifications than it is for masses and distortion. Once the areas of possible abnormality have been identified, the radiologist must decide whether the patient needs to return for additional imaging.

In a prospective study on the effects of CAD, radiologist recall rate changed slightly (from 6.5% to 7.7%), and there was a 19.5% increase in the number of cancers detected. Cancers were detected at an earlier stage: The percentage of stage 0 and stage 1 malignancies detected increased from 73% to 78%.

Notes

Challenge

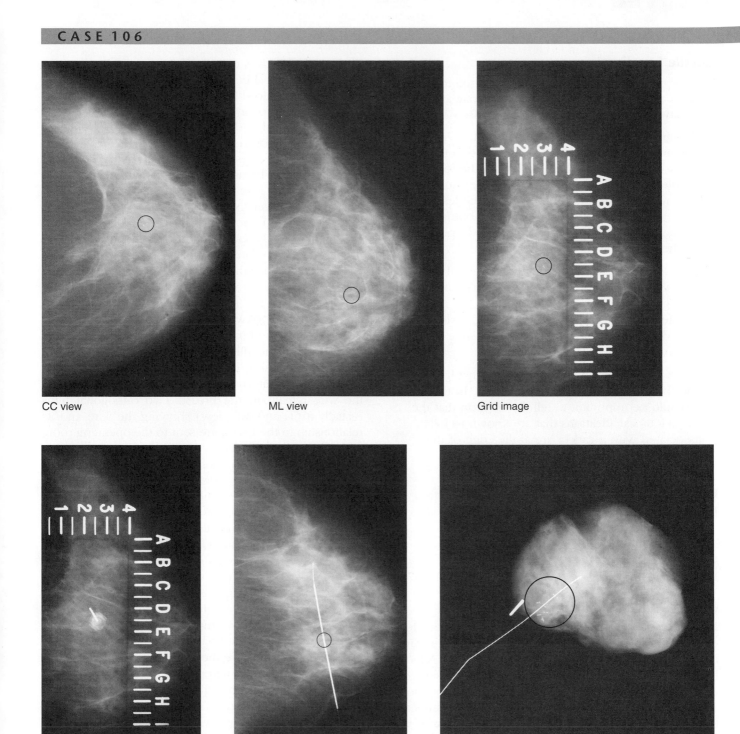

CC view

ML view

Grid image

After needle placed

ML view to show needle in lesion

Specimen

1. This patient has had an 11-gauge stereotactic core biopsy that yielded DCIS, and there are residual calcifications in the right central breast for which a needle localization was recommended. What is the likelihood that the stereotactic core biopsy "understaged" the lesion and there is actually invasive carcinoma?

2. The calcifications are circled. Using an alphanumeric grid for the needle localization, how would you ask the technologist to position the patient?

3. What gauge and type of needle is used for this procedure? What images are sent with the patient to the operating room?

4. Is a specimen radiograph necessary? What is important to note about this specimen when talking to the surgeon?

Needle Localization

1. Approximately 11% of lesions determined to be DCIS at 11-gauge stereotactic core biopsy are found to have an invasive component at excision.

2. The grid device should be placed so that the grid opening is over the closest skin surface to the site of the calcifications. Therefore, when the localizing needle is inserted through the skin, the shortest distance (and the shortest needle) to the lesion is chosen. In this case, the patient should be placed in the reverse CC position with the grid opening on the inferior aspect of the breast.

3. A 20- or 21-gauge needle that has a central open bore that accommodates a hookwire. The two orthogonal images (usually CC and ML) of the needle and/or wire placement with the lesion circled go with the patient to the operating room to serve as a "map" for the surgeon.

4. Yes, a specimen is needed to confirm that the lesion and the hookwire have been removed. In this case, it would be important to tell the surgeon that the suspicious calcifications that are known to be associated with a cancer are at the edge of the specimen.

Reference

Liberman L: Percutaneous image-guided core breast biopsy, *Radiol Clin North Am* 40:483–500, 2002.

Cross-Reference

Ikeda, *Breast Imaging: THE REQUISITES*, pp 164–167.

Comment

Needle localization procedures are performed less often today than in previous years due to the wide acceptance of percutaneous core biopsies. Needle localizations are necessary to accurately guide a surgeon to an area that is nonpalpable and requires excision. To expedite the localization on the day of the surgery, the lesion should have been entirely worked up (magnifications, if needed, to establish the extent of a lesion) and triangulated on orthogonal imaging. Needle localization may be performed under either ultrasound or radiographic guidance. The selection of the guiding modality should be based on the ease of seeing the lesion. Calcifications are generally localized under mammographic guidance and masses are usually localized with ultrasound guidance.

For a mammographically guided needle localization, the most important step is positioning the patient so that the skin entry site for placement of the localizing needle and hookwire is from the closest skin surface.

The needle length is chosen by measuring the distance from the closest skin surface to the site of the lesion. The patient is placed in compression with the alphanumeric grid open over the appropriate skin surface. The patient is imaged and the coordinates at the center of the lesion are chosen (in this case, D1/4, 2½). The skin is cleansed and anesthetized and then the needle is placed into the breast. To ensure that the needle is placed into the lesion, an image of the needle hub superimposed over the shaft of the needle is obtained. The patient is removed from compression and an orthogonal view is obtained showing the position of the tip of the needle relative to the lesion. The needle depth is adjusted so that the tip of the needle is at or just beyond the lesion. (In this case, the needle was placed slightly deep to the lesion and had to be withdrawn slightly.) The hookwire is then placed through the needle and secured in the breast tissue. Some surgeons prefer that the needle be kept in the breast to aid in localizing the lesion in the operating room; other surgeons prefer that the needle be removed and only the wire remain in the breast. Two orthogonal films (usually a CC and ML view) showing the wire and its relationship to the lesion are sent to the operating room with the lesion circled.

The specimen radiograph is an essential component of the radiographically needle localization procedure. It is imperative that the radiologist review the specimen to ensure that the lesion has been removed (or sampled, in some cases). If a needle localization is performed under ultrasound guidance, an ultrasound of the specimen may be necessary to confirm that the lesion has been removed if it is not evident on the radiograph of the specimen. The surgeon is notified of the specimen radiograph findings, and if the lesion has not been removed or adequately sampled, the surgeon should be directed to obtain more tissue. In this case, the surgeon had intended to remove the entire area of calcifications and also obtain clean margins for a lumpectomy. The specimen radiograph reveals that the calcifications are at the edge of the tissue. The surgeon was directed to obtain more tissue from where the "clipped" edge of the specimen came from. This communication from the radiologist assists the surgeon in obtaining clean margins and reducing the likelihood of reexcision.

Notes

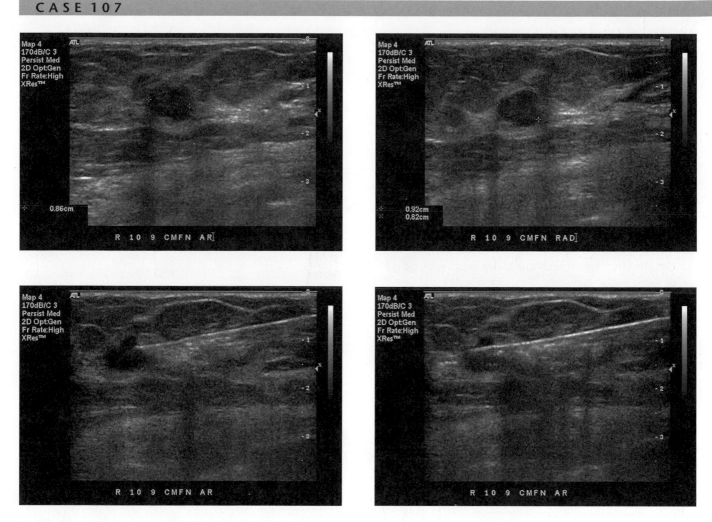

1. Describe the ultrasound findings in the first two images.

2. Describe the sequence of events in the images, all obtained within 1 minute.

3. What is the appropriate needle orientation with respect to the chest wall?

4. How many samples should be taken with this 14-gauge biopsy device?

Ultrasound-Guided Core Biopsy

1. There is a solid mass in the breast with the benign features of four gentle lobulations, thin capsule, and no shadowing. However, it is rounded rather than oblong in shape, and it is hypoechoic to surrounding fat, which are more suspicious findings. Since the features are not completely benign, biopsy was recommended.

2. This is an ultrasound-guided core biopsy using an automated 14-guage device.

3. The biopsy needle should stay close to parallel to the chest wall to avoid entering the muscle or pleura.

4. Usually, five specimens are taken with a 14-gauge device.

References

Liberman L: Percutaneous imaging-guided core breast biopsy: State of the art at the millennium, *Am J Roentgenol* 174:1191–1199, 2000.

Mainiero MB, Gareen IF, Bird CE, Smith W, Cobb C, Schepps B: Preferential use of sonographically guided biopsy to minimize patient discomfort and procedure time in a percutaneous image-guided breast biopsy program, *J Ultrasound Med* 21(11):1221–1226, 2002.

Parker SH, Jobe WE, Dennis MA, et al.: US-guided automated large-core breast biopsy, *Radiology* 187:507–511, 1993.

Cross-Reference

Ikeda, *Breast Imaging: THE REQUISITES*, p 173.

Comment

Image-guided core needle biopsy is the preferred method for sampling palpable and nonpalpable masses and calcifications in the breast. Core biopsy provides a better sampling of the lesion compared to fine needle aspiration biopsy. Core biopsy samples are histologic rather than cytologic specimens. There is a greater volume of material, with more complete sampling of the lesion. In fine needle aspiration, cells are removed from the lesion and smeared on a slide. The cytopathologist reads for the presence or absence of malignant cells but cannot differentiate *in situ* from invasive disease.

Core biopsies can be directed by mammography (stereotactic), ultrasound, or MRI. Of the three, ultrasound is usually the fastest method, least expensive, and easier for the patient because the patient does not have to hold completely still and is generally more comfortable. Ultrasound allows for access to any part of the breast and axilla, does not use ionizing radiation or compression, and is the only method to allow real-time visualization of the biopsy procedure.

Compared to surgical biopsy, image-guided biopsy is less expensive, less invasive, causes little to no scarring, and has fewer complications. Complications may include hematoma and infection, which occur in less than 1 in 1000 biopsies, according to published reports.

If the result of the biopsy is benign with no atypia, surgery is not necessary. If the result of the biopsy is malignant, fewer surgical procedures are needed because the patient can proceed to definitive surgery with sentinel node biopsy. However, most breast lesions sampled with image-guided biopsy are benign (approximately 70–80%).

This patient's lesion was malignant—an invasive ductal cancer, not otherwise specified.

Notes

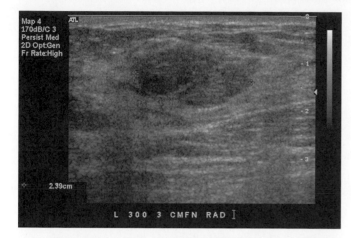

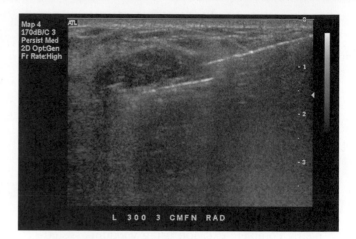

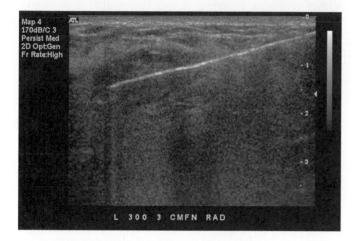

1. Describe the ultrasound finding.

2. Is biopsy indicated?

3. Describe the needle procedure being performed.

4. Can masses be excised using a core technique?

Ultrasound-Guided Vacuum-Assisted Core Biopsy

1. There is an oval, circumscribed solid mass with gentle lobulations, wider than tall, with no posterior shadowing, isoechoic to fat, all characteristic of a probably benign mass.

2. Biopsy can be performed at the patient's discretion.

3. This is a vacuum-assisted core biopsy. The needle is placed into the lesion, the chamber in the needle opens (middle image), and then the core cutting sleeve cuts the core of tissue (third image).

4. A smaller mass (<1.5 cm) has the likelihood of nearly complete excision using vacuum-assisted core biopsy. Larger masses such as this one are usually not completed excised. If a mass is malignant on core biopsy, surgical excision is still necessary.

References

March DE, Coughlin BF, Barham RB, Goulart RA, Klein SV, Bur ME, Frank JL, Makari-Judson G: Breast masses: Removal of all US evidence during biopsy by using a handheld vacuum-assisted device—Initial experience, *Radiology* 227:549–555, 2003.

Parker SH, Jobe WE, Dennis MA, Stavros AT, Johnson KK, Yakes WF, Truell JE, Price JG, Kortz AB, Clark DG: US-guided automated large-core breast biopsy, *Radiology* 187:507, 1993.

Parker SH, Klaus AJ, McWey PJ, Schilling KJ, Cupples TE, Duchesne N, Guenin MA, Harness JK: Sonographically guided directional vacuum-assisted breast biopsy using a handheld device, *Am J Roentgenol* 177:405–408, 2001.

Philpotts LE, Hooley RJ, Lee CH: Comparison of automated versus vacuum-assisted biopsy methods for sonographically guided core biopsy of the breast, *Am J Roentgenol* 180(2):347–351, 2003.

Simon JR, Kalbhen CL, Cooper RA, Flisak ME: Accuracy and complication rates of US-guided vacuum-assisted core breast biopsy: Initial results, *Radiology* 215:694, 2000.

Cross-Reference

Ikeda, *Breast Imaging: THE REQUISITES*, p 177.

Comment

Image-guided core biopsy is a safe, less costly alternative to surgical excisional biopsy. Histopathology diagnosis is reliable, and the procedure is less traumatic than surgery. The relatively small amount of tissue retrieved at core biopsy may underestimate the severity of the lesion. The introduction of larger bore needles with vacuum assistance was intended to obtain more tissue at biopsy to ensure a more accurate diagnosis. The larger bore needles may also completely remove a small lesion (percutaneous excision).

The vacuum-assisted biopsy is now the standard for stereotactically guided biopsy; however, it is less well established for ultrasound-guided biopsy. Previously, the 14-gauge spring-loaded core needle was the standard technology for both methods. The type of lesion sampled with stereotactic guidance is different from the lesion sampled using ultrasound guidance. Stereotactic biopsy is used primarily for calcifications and for small, deep masses because these lesions are not seen well on ultrasound. Lesions that are seen well on ultrasound are sampled preferentially with ultrasound because it allows real-time imaging, is quicker, and is more comfortable for the patient. Sampling of calcifications requires more core specimens than a mass to ensure that the lesion is adequately sampled so that underestimation of malignancy occurs less often.

Are there similar benefits to using a large core biopsy device when sampling masses using ultrasound? When the 11-gauge device was introduced, merits of this needle size over the 14-gauge included a decrease in the underestimation of malignancy, a decrease in sampling error (particularly in small, deep lesions difficult to see on ultrasound), and a decrease in the rebiopsy rate, particularly of fibroadenomas that increase in size after needle core biopsy. Fewer cores are needed to obtain the same volume of sampling since the gauge is larger; thus, the biopsy may be quicker with the larger gauge needles. Several studies have shown that the complication rates of the 14-gauge and the 11-gauge device are similar.

Notes

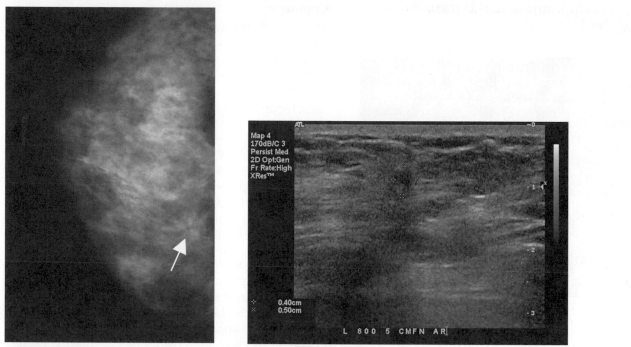

CC view of left breast

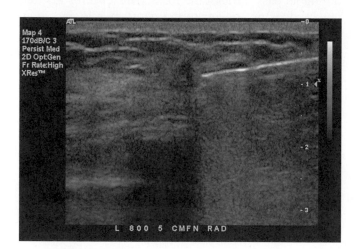

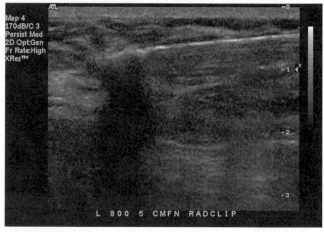

US of left 8:00 region

1. Describe the mammographic abnormality on this left CC view at the arrow.

2. Are spot compression views needed, or should ultrasound be used next?

3. Does the mass seen on ultrasound correspond with the mammographic finding?

4. Should biopsy be performed with ultrasound or with mammographic guidance?

Cancer on Mammogram and Ultrasound— Biopsy under Ultrasound

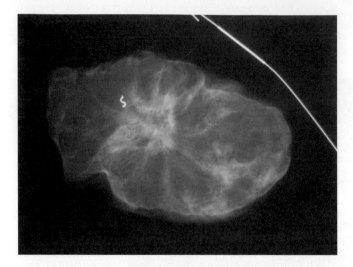

1. There is architectural distortion in the medial left breast.

2. Spot compression views can be useful to ensure that the architectural distortion persists and is not due to overlapping normal glandular elements. Additional views may also be needed to triangulate the location of the distortion, and they are most useful before using ultrasound. Once the lesion has been shown to persist and its location identified, ultrasound is performed.

3. The size, location, and appearance of the mass match on mammography and ultrasound. The mass is in the lower inner left breast at 8 o'clock.

4. If the mass is seen on both mammogram and ultrasound, it is usually easier to biopsy using ultrasound guidance.

References

Fishman JE, Milikowski C, Ramsinghani R, Velasquez MV, Aviram G: US-guided core-needle biopsy of the breast: How many specimens are necessary? *Radiology* 226(3):779–782, 2003.

Parker SH, Burbank F, Jackman RJ, Aucreman CJ, Cardenosa G, Cink TM, Coscia JL Jr, Eklund GW, Evans WP 3rd, Garver PR: Percutaneous large-core breast biopsy: A multi-institutional study, *Radiology* 193:359–364, 1994.

Cross-Reference

Ikeda, *Breast Imaging: THE REQUISITES*, p 173.

Comment

This patient had a screening exam, one view of which is shown. Subtle architectural distortion was noted on the CC view in the medial left breast. Spot compression views failed to efface the distortion, and ultrasound was performed.

Ultrasound is a useful exam in the patient with a mammographic abnormality. In this patient, a small mass was seen in the medial breast, which corresponded well with the location and size of the mammographic distortion. The mass has a suspicious appearance on ultrasound: It is taller than wide, hypoechoic, with a thick, irregular echogenic rim and posterior acoustic shadowing.

Biopsy can be performed with ultrasound guidance in this patient. The technique involves marking the skin entry location approximately 4 cm from the lesion. This distance from the lesion will be dependent on the depth of the mass in the breast: Shallower masses can be approached at a closer location, whereas deeper lesions will need to be approached from a greater distance. The reason for this is that the biopsy needle must be parallel to the chest wall, or as close to parallel as possible, during its pass through the mass. This ensures that the needle does not penetrate the chest muscle and lung. In this example, the needle biopsy device is a spring-loaded 14-gauge device, and the images show the needle at the edge of the lesion and after it is fired through the lesion. Five passes are usually made through the lesion when using a 14-gauge device.

A clip can be placed at the site of biopsy. This is a useful procedure after biopsy if the mammographic finding is subtle because it makes it easier to locate the mass at the time of surgery. Specimen radiograph is shown, with the S-shaped clip adjacent to the mass. Histopathology was a low-grade invasive ductal carcinoma.

Notes

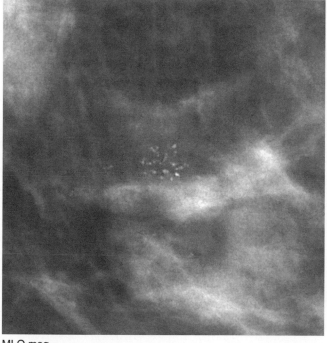

MLO mag

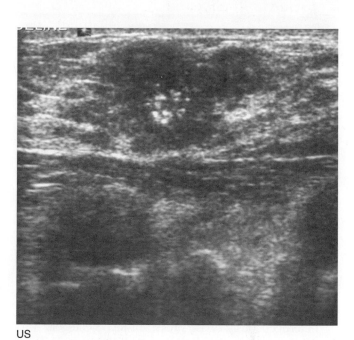

US

1. Describe the mammographic findings and give a BI-RADS category.

2. Describe the ultrasound findings and give a BI-RADS category.

3. Does the combination of imaging findings from the ultrasound and mammogram suggest a histology?

4. What type of biopsy would you recommend in this case? Why?

Calcifications on Ultrasound

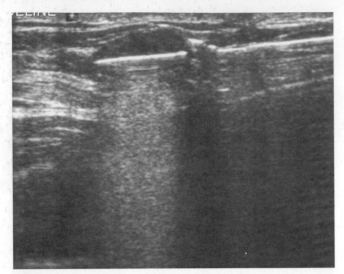

US core

1. There is a cluster of pleomorphic calcifications in this heterogeneously dense breast. BI-RADS category 4.

2. On ultrasound, there is a hypoechoic irregular mass that contains calcifications. The hypoechoic mass is larger that the area of calcifications seen mammographically, BI-RADS category 5.

3. The hypoechoic irregular mass suggests that there is an invasive component of cancer associated with the mammographically detected cluster of suspicious calcifications.

4. In this case, stereotactic or ultrasound-guided core biopsy could be performed. However, ultrasound-guided biopsy would be better able to target the solid mass, which is probably the invasive component of this lesion.

Reference

Berg WA, Gilbreath PL: Multicentric and multifocal cancer: Whole breast ultrasound in preoperative evaluation, *Radiology* 214:59–66, 2000.

Cross-Reference

Ikeda, *Breast Imaging: THE REQUISITES*, p 149.

Comment

This patient has a small cluster of calcifications seen in an area of the breast that is heterogeneously dense mammographically; no distortion or mass are seen. The calcifications are suspicious, and based on the mammographic appearance, the patient most likely has at least DCIS. In this case, ultrasound evaluation provides additional information. The ultrasound shows an unsuspected mass that is associated with the calcifications.

The irregular and hypoechoic mass is highly suspicious for an invasive component of malignancy. Although the cluster of calcifications could be biopsied with stereotactic guidance, ultrasound-guided core biopsy could better target the area of highest concern—the irregular mass. Invasive ductal carcinoma with a component of high-grade DCIS was found histologically.

Ultrasound is much better at detecting invasive carcinomas than finding *in situ* carcinomas. Ultrasound may occasionally show high-grade DCIS associated with very course calcifications in a hypoechoic area or in a hypoechoic dilated duct, but usually this area is first detected mammographically. In this case, the mammographic findings were suspicious, but the addition of the irregular mass seen on ultrasound increased the degree of concern, bringing it to a BI-RADS category 5. The combination of the two imaging studies in this patient provided a more accurate assessment of disease.

Notes

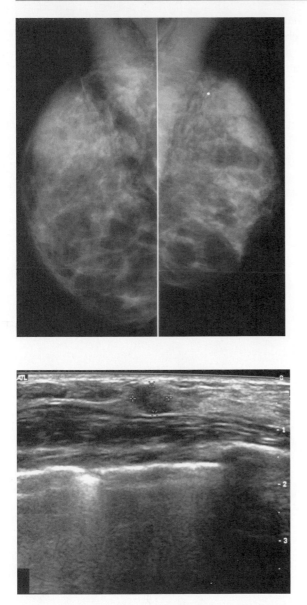

1. This patient underwent right breast conservation therapy for cancer 7 years ago and now notes a palpable mass in the right breast. What is your first diagnostic exam?

2. What is done as the second exam?

3. Can this mass be approached for image-guided biopsy?

4. Would you use stereotactic or ultrasound-guided biopsy?

Core Biopsy of Small Superficial Mass (Recurrence)

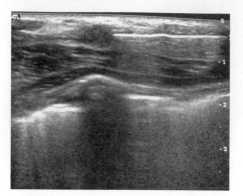

1. Bilateral mammogram with marker over the area of concern.

2. Ultrasound of the palpable finding.

3. Yes, this mass can be sampled using imaging guidance.

4. Since the mass is not seen on mammogram, but is seen on ultrasound, use ultrasound to biopsy.

References

Liberman L, Ernberg LA, Heerdt A, Zakowski MF, Morris EA, LaTrenta LR, Abramson AF, Dershaw DD: Palpable breast masses: Is there a role for percutaneous imaging-guided core biopsy? *Am J Roentgenol* 175(3):779–787, 2000.

Parker SH, Burbank F: A practical approach to minimally invasive breast biopsy, *Radiology* 200:11–20, 1996.

Cross-Reference

Ikeda, *Breast Imaging: THE REQUISITES*, pp 173, 233.

Comment

An ipsilateral palpable mass in a patient who has undergone breast conservation therapy is suspicious for recurrence. Biopsy should be performed. If the pathology of the new mass in the conserved breast is malignant, mastectomy may be recommended. However, if the palpable finding in this premenopausal patient is benign, such as fibroadenoma, then no surgical management may be needed.

This core biopsy is somewhat challenging because of the location of the mass—in the axillary tail of the breast. Care must be taken so that the biopsy needle stays parallel to the chest wall and does not angle toward the chest muscle and the lung. In order to keep the needle parallel, the skin entry point of the needle must be several centimeters away from the tumor site. This allows room to place the needle through the skin on a shallow angle. The needle is then aligned parallel to the chest wall as it enters the mass. The path of the needle must be carefully observed on ultrasound the entire time the needle is in the breast.

Notes

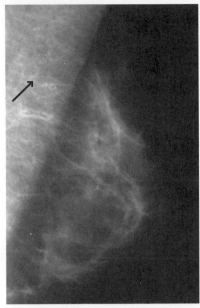

Initial right MLO

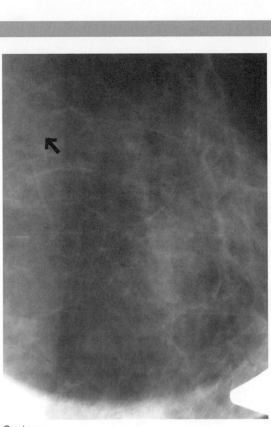

Spot mag

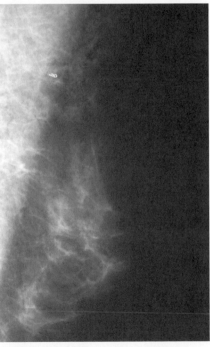

Postbiopsy with clip

1. Describe the findings in the first image.

2. A spot magnification view is shown. What should be done next? What is the BI-RADS category and recommendation?

3. Is this an area that can be biopsied successfully using the stereotactic approach?

4. If the stereotactic biopsy is not successful, can the patient be followed with 6-month mammogram?

Difficult Stereotactic Biopsy Cases—Calcifications in the Axillary Tail of the Breast

1. There is a grouping of microcalcifications in the upper posterior breast, overlying the pectoral muscle.

2. Most of the calcifications are punctuate and round, but there are several faint, amorphous forms. Biopsy is indicated for this cluster of indeterminate calcifications. BI-RADS category 4.

3. The axillary tail of the breast may be difficult to target for stereotactic biopsy and may require special positioning of the patient.

4. If stereotactic needle biopsy is not successful, the patient must be sent for surgical excisional biopsy.

Reference

Jackman RJ, Marzoni FA Jr: Stereotactic histologic biopsy with patients prone: Technical feasibility in 98% of mammographically detected lesions, *Am J Roentgenol* 180:785–794, 2003.

Cross-Reference

Ikeda, *Breast Imaging: THE REQUISITES*, p 177.

Comment

In a paper published in 2003, nearly 2000 stereotactic biopsies and reasons for incomplete and canceled studies were reviewed. When biopsies were canceled for technical reasons, the majority were canceled because the lesion was too close to the chest wall.

Lesions close to the chest wall and in the axillary tail are difficult to position for the mammogram and difficult to position in the stereotactic window for biopsy. However, there are maneuvers that can be used to better visualize posterior lesions so that they can be sampled stereotactically.

The breast should be pulled, gently but firmly, as completely as possible down through the opening in the stereotactic table. The patient should be encouraged to relax the chest muscles as much as possible. If the lesion cannot be seen, the patient's arm can be placed through the breast opening, which drops more of the axillary area into position for biopsy. The patient can also be rolled into a slightly decubitus position, with the side of interest down.

Calcifications in the axillary tail may be easier to biopsy from the MLO or mediolateral approach rather than the CC approach. From the lateral approach, the calcifications will be closer to the skin.

The post biopsy mammogram demonstrates the clip at the site where the calcifications had been present.

In this patient, histopathology of the calcifications on biopsy was benign.

Notes

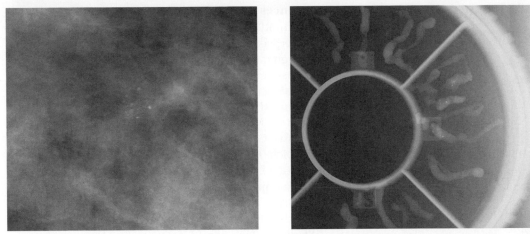

Specimen radiograph

A spot magnification view shows a cluster of pleomorphic calcifications. Stereotactic core biopsy was requested.

1. What technical issues might limit the ability to biopsy lesions by stereotactic core biopsy?

2. The calcifications were removed entirely by stereotactic core. What is needed next?

3. The result from the core was atypical ductal hyperplasia (ADH). What is the follow-up recommendation and why?

4. Does the fact that the calcifications were entirely removed improve the concordance between the stereotactic core histology and the final excisional biopsy histology?

Atypical Ductal Hyperplasia

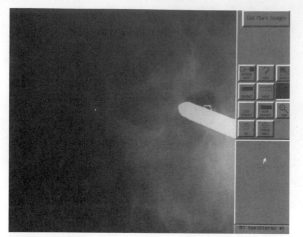

Needle with clip

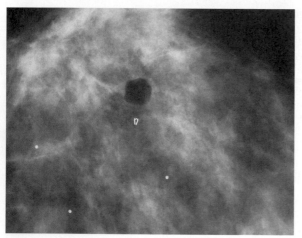

Post bx cavity

1. Stereotactic core biopsy may not be possible if the calcifications are not visible (i.e., too close to the chest wall or too far posterior in the axillary tail) or if the breast is too thin to accommodate the needle (usually difficult if the breast is less that 2 cm thick under compression).

2. A clip should be left at the site of biopsy and two orthogonal mammographic views should be obtained to confirm the biopsy site, any residual lesion, and the placement of the clip relative to the biopsy site.

3. Exicisional biopsy because the lesion may represent an understaging. More tissue may show that there is actually DCIS associated with the calcifications.

4. Yes, there is better concordance, but an excision is still needed to ensure there is not a more significant lesion such as DCIS. In this case, DCIS was found at excision.

References

Jackman RJ, Birdwell RL, Ikeda DM: Atypical ductal hyperplasia: Can some lesions be defined as probably benign after stereotactic 11-gauge vacuum-assisted biopsy, eliminating the recommendation for surgical excision? *Radiology* 224:548–554, 2002.

Jackman RJ, Burbank F, Parker SH, Evans WP III, Lechner MC, Richardson TR, Smid AA, Borofsky HB, Lee CH, Goldstein HM, Schilling KJ, Wray AB, Brem RF, Helbich TH, Lehrer DE, Adler SJ: Stereotactic breast biopsy of nonpalpable lesions: Determinants of ductal carcinoma in situ underestimation rates, *Radiology* 218:497, 2001.

Lomoschitz FM, Helbich TH, Rudas M, Pfarl G, Linnau KF, Stadler A, Jackman RJ: Stereotactic 11-gauge vacuum-assisted breast biopsy: Influence of number of specimens on diagnostic accuracy, *Radiology* 232:897–903, 2004.

Cross-Reference

Ikeda, *Breast Imaging: THE REQUISITES*, pp 183–184.

Comment

ADH is in the spectrum of hyperplastic changes that range from usual ductal hyperplasia to DCIS. ADH is found in approximately 5% of all biopsies performed for any type of calcifications but is frequently found associated with regional amorphous calcifications (approximately 20%). In this case, the calcifications were a very focal cluster of heterogeneous and pleomorphic calcifications and the suspicion level was relatively high that the lesion was DCIS.

ADH diagnosed by core biopsy should always undergo surgical excisional biopsy due to the high incidence of histologic underestimation of DCIS. Using an 11-guage vacuum-assisted core needle, there is an approximately 25% underestimation of malignancy when ADH is the diagnosis. Lesions that undergo core biopsies and are interpreted as ADH demonstrate various histologies on excision, including fibrocystic change, ADH, DCIS, and invasive ductal carcinoma.

In this case, the calcifications appear to have been removed entirely on core biopsy. A small clip marks the site of biopsy so that if excision is needed, the area is easily localized. However, complete removal of all the mammographic evidence of the calcifications at core biopsy does not obviate the need for excision. A few studies have shown that the more calcifications that can be removed at core biopsy, the higher the concordance at excision. However, the goal of stereotactic core biopsy is not complete removal but, rather, adequate sampling of the lesion. The final diagnosis was low-grade DCIS.

Notes

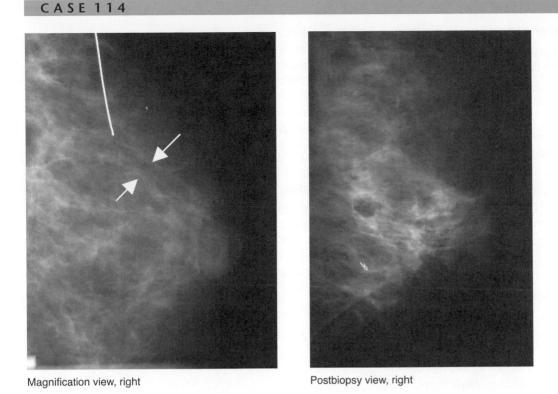

Magnification view, right   Postbiopsy view, right

1. This patient is 1-year postlumpectomy and radiation therapy for DCIS, now with this magnification view of the lumpectomy site. What is your interpretation of the findings at the arrows? What is the BI-RADS category?

2. What is in your differential diagnosis?

3. Stereotactic core biopsy was performed, showing DCIS, and a clip was placed. What is your interpretation of the second image?

4. What must be included in the biopsy procedure report?

Clip Displacement after Stereotactic Biopsy

1. There are microcalcifications anterior and inferior to the lumpectomy site. BI-RADS 4: biopsy recommended.

2. The calcifications may represent recurrence or inadequate resection of cancer performed 1 year prior. They may also represent benign dystrophic calcifications developing after surgery and radiation therapy.

3. The air-filled biopsy cavity is at the site where the calcifications had been. There are no residual calcifications. The clip is not at the biopsy cavity but is inferiorly displaced.

4. The clip displaced 1.5 mm inferior to biopsy site. The true location of the disease is not indicated by the clip. This must be communicated to the surgeon.

References

Birdwell RL, Jackman RJ: Clip or marker migration 5–10 weeks after stereotactic 11-gauge vacuum-assisted breast biopsy: Report of two cases, *Radiology* 229(2): 541–544, 2003.

Esserman LE, Cura MA, DaCosta D: Recognizing pitfalls in early and late migration of clip markers after imaging-guided directional vacuum-assisted biopsy, *RadioGraphics* 24(1):147–156, 2004.

Philpotts LE, Lee CH: Clip migration after 11-gauge vacuum-assisted stereotactic biopsy: Case report, *Radiology* 222:794–796, 2002.

Cross-Reference

Ikeda, *Breast Imaging: THE REQUISITES*, p 181.

Comment

This 52-year-old patient was initially diagnosed with developing suspicious microcalcifications on routine mammogram. She underwent stereotactic needle core biopsy of the microcalcifications, which showed DCIS. Excisional biopsy showed DCIS associated with microcalcifications. Her surgical margins were clear of disease. She underwent radiation therapy.

Fifteen months later, follow-up mammogram was performed. Magnification views of the lumpectomy site were performed. These views demonstrated that microcalcifications had developed since the prior exam. Stereotactic needle core biopsy was performed and showed DCIS with associated microcalcifications. A clip was placed at the time of biopsy through the 11-gauge stereotactic biopsy device.

A two-view mammogram of the right breast was performed after the biopsy to document the site of biopsy, to determine if any calcifications remain, and to check the position of the clip. On this exam, the clip was displaced 1.5 cm inferior to the air-filled biopsy cavity.

Displacement of the clip following biopsy is a known complication of stereotactic biopsy with clip placement. This displacement needs to be communicated to the surgeon. No residual calcifications are present in the breast to denote the location of disease. The clip is placed to mark the exact site of the biopsy. If the displacement away from the disease site is not discussed, when the patient returns for excisional biopsy, the clip will be used to localize the site of disease and the residual cancer will be missed. In this case, the clip displacement was communicated to the surgeon, and the correct area was excised. The postsurgery mammogram may show the displaced biopsy clip in the breast. This needs to be recognized on the mammogram and is not to be interpreted as a failure to excise the correct area.

Notes

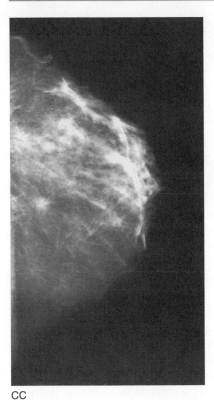

CC

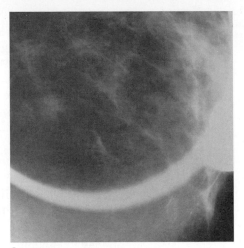

Spot mag

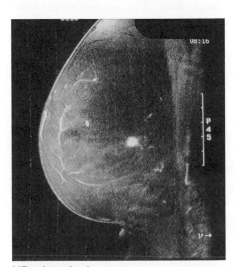

MR subtraction image

1. The right cranial caudad view shows a new focal asymmetry seen only on the CC view. What additional imaging is recommended?

2. A spot magnification view suggests that the small asymmetry is a spiculated mass. Orthogonal mammographic views were performed but no definite lesion was seen. Focused ultrasound from the superior and inferior central (12 and 6 o'clock sites) also failed to localize a mass. What might the next step be?

3. MRI subtraction image shows an irregular, avidly enhancing mass deep in the central breast. What is the next recommendation?

4. An MRI-guided needle localization was performed. Is a specimen radiograph necessary?

MRI Needle Localization

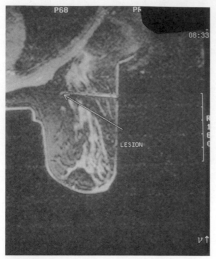

MR needle

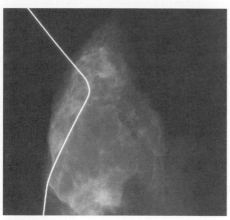

Specimen

1. The next step in working up this patient would be to obtain a straight lateral or rolled CC view to try to triangulate the mass.

2. Although ultrasound and orthogonal mammographic views fail to show a lesion, the concern level is still high due to the spiculated appearance of the mass on the cranial caudad spot magnification view. An MRI was obtained for further evaluation.

3. A core biopsy or needle localization under MRI guidance was recommended.

4. MRI shows that the needle for localization is correctly placed and a wire was then left to guide the excisional biopsy. Specimen radiographs are recommended; however, it may be difficult to find the mass. In this case, the mass is surrounded by fat and is evident on the specimen. If an MRI core is performed, a clip should be left to mark the biopsy site.

Reference

Orel SG, Schnall MD: MR imaging of the breast for the detection, diagnosis, and staging of breast cancer, *Radiology* 220:13–30, 2001.

Cross-Reference

Ikeda, *Breast Imaging: THE REQUISITES*, pp 217–221.

Comment

This case is a diagnostic dilemma. A new focal asymmetry is visualized on the cranial caudad view and persists on spot magnification. The magnification view suggests that the margin of the small mass is spiculated. Despite additional rolled cranial caudad views, straight lateral mammographic views, and focused ultrasound, the exact location of this mass is not known. Although a stereotactic core biopsy could be performed in the cranial caudal projection, an MRI was recommended. The MRI shows a highly suspicious mass with irregular margins in the central breast that corresponds in size with the mammmographic finding. The mass shows avid enhancement with rapid washout of gadolinium on delayed imaging, which is also a suspicious finding.

A needle localization for excisional biopsy was performed under MRI guidance. A core biopsy could also have been performed with the appropriate MRI-compatible equipment. One technique used for MRI needle localization is to use a special lateral compression plate that has multiple holes drilled to allow the localizing needle to enter the lateral breast. Just as with mammographically guided needle localizations, when MRI-guided needle localizations are performed, it is important to ensure that the needle and hookwire are in the correct location in the breast. Confirmation is performed with MRI before the patient is released from compression. A two-view mammogram is also performed to show the location of the wire in the breast, even if the lesion was not visible previously mammographically. Although a specimen image cannot be obtained with MRI, a mammographic specimen radiograph is performed. In this case, a small spiculated mass was visualized at the edge of the mammographic specimen; a small 6-mm invasive ductal carcinoma was seen histologically.

Notes

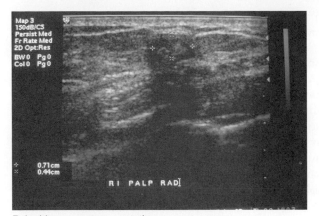

Palpable mass at presentation

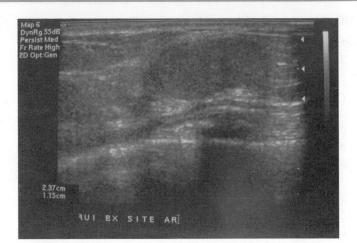

US 6 months later

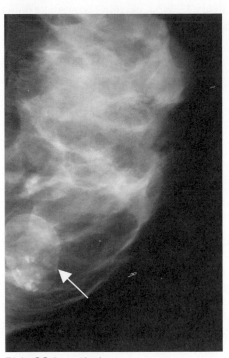

Right CC 6 months later

1. This patient presents with a palpable mass in her third trimester of pregnancy. What is the most likely diagnosis?

2. What are the options for further evaluation?

3. The patient complains of a persistent lump, larger than the original lump, 6 months later at the biopsy site. What is in your differential diagnosis?

4. What is your diagnosis of the mammogram of the biopsy site taken after delivery?

Milk Fistula—Galactocele: Complication of Core Biopsy during Lactation

1. This is a solid mass, most likely a benign lesion such as lactating adenoma or fibroadenoma.

2. Core biopsy can be performed during pregnancy. This mass has benign features of oval shape, circumscribed margin, hypoechoic echotexture, and abrupt interface with surrounding tissue, and it could be followed closely with ultrasound. This patient demanded biopsy.

3. The most common complication is hematoma, but this would not commonly be seen 6 months after biopsy. A milk fistula can occur in this population after either needle biopsy or excisional biopsy.

4. The mammogram shows a mixed-density, partially lucent mass, consistent with a galactocele resulting from milk fistula.

References

Parker SH, Stavros AT, Dennis MA: Needle biopsy techniques, *Radiol Clin North Am* 33:1171–1186, 1995.

Schackmuth EM, Harlow CL, Norton LW: Milk fistula: A complication after core breast biopsy, *Am J Roentgenol* 161:961–962, 1993.

Sumkin JH, Perrone AM, Harris KM, Nath ME, Amortegui AJ, Weinstein BJ: Lactating adenoma: US features and literature review, *Radiology* 206:271–274, 1998.

Cross-Reference

Ikeda, *Breast Imaging: THE REQUISITES*, pp 185, 288.

Comment

This patient presented with a palpable mass in the right breast. Ultrasound was performed as the initial exam because she was in the third trimester of pregnancy at the time of detection of the mass. A needle core biopsy of the palpable mass in the right upper inner breast was performed, and histology of the mass was lactating adenoma. No immediate complications were seen. Several weeks after the biopsy, the patient returned with a palpable mass, larger than the original palpable finding. Ultrasound of the new finding showed a well-circumscribed oval mass consistent with a complex cyst, likely galactocele resulting from milk fistula. The patient was reassured that this should resolve spontaneously, and she was followed by ultrasound. The mass decreased in size and then resolved completely after several months.

The most common palpable masses in pregnant and lactating women are lactating adenomas and fibroadenomas; lactating adenomas represent 70% of masses undergoing biopsy in this population. A lactating adenoma is most often seen on ultrasound as an oval, hypoechoic mass, well circumscribed, parallel to the chest wall. However, a lactating adenoma can have a more suspicious appearance, with shadowing and irregular margins, making malignancy more difficult to exclude.

Although the mass had benign features on ultrasound exam, this patient was concerned about the possibility of malignancy and requested biopsy. This is an acceptable approach in the probably benign lesion, BI-RADS 3. Any intervention in the breast carries a possibility of complications, although complications of needle core biopsy are unusual (approximately 1 or 2% in many published series). The most common complications are hematoma and infection. An additional complication that can occur in the third trimester of pregnancy or during lactation is the milk fistula. Damage to the ducts by the needle causes leaking of duct contents (milk) into the biopsy cavity.

Notes

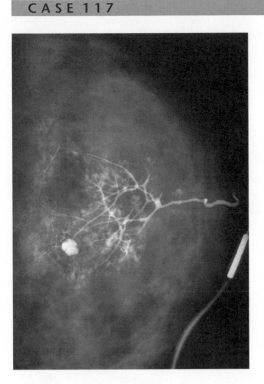

1. This patient presents with a clear yellow, spontaneous discharge from one opening of the right nipple. What is your interpretation of this galactogram?

2. Why is contrast seen in rounded areas adjacent to the ducts?

3. Is this considered contrast extravasation?

4. What is the next step?

Normal Galactogram

1. This is a normal galactogram.

2. Contrast has entered into lobules.

3. No. Extravasation is caused by rupture of the duct, causing the contrast to pool outside the ruptured duct. The rounded areas are due to filling of the lobules.

4. This galactogram does not give the etiology of the unilateral spontaneous discharge. A follow-up galactogram should be performed. It is likely that the wrong duct was entered. Another alternative would be to refer the patient to a surgeon for evaluation or to perform MRI.

References

Cardenosa G, Doudna C, Eklund GW: Ductography of the breast: Technique and findings, *Am J Roentgenol* 162:1081–1087, 1994.

Slawson SH, Johnson BA: Ductography: How to and what if? *RadioGraphics* 21(1):133–150, 2001.

Cross-Reference

Ikeda, *Breast Imaging: THE REQUISITES*, pp 293–294.

Comment

This is an example of a galactogram of a normal duct. There are no suspicious features. In this normal exam, the ducts are thin, with smooth walls, regular branching, and no filling defects. Abnormal ducts are enlarged and may have irregular duct walls, abrupt termination of ducts, and filling defects.

This example shows the effect of maximal pressure exerted during the galactogram. The contrast has entered the lobules, including one cyst in communication with the duct. The rounded areas of contrast outside the ducts in this patient represent contrast that has entered the lobules, called "lobular blush." This is not extravasation, which occurs when the cannula perforates the side wall of the duct and a pool of contrast occurs outside the duct lumen and which is to be avoided.

Galactography is performed when there is a clinically suspicious discharge, which is a unilateral, spontaneous, clear, yellow, pink, or bloody discharge. Patients with this type of discharge may frequently have an underlying cancer (up to 33%). Benign causes of discharge, such as papilloma, are more common than malignancy. It is not necessary to perform galactography for nipple discharge that is bilateral, nonspontaneous, occurring in multiple duct orifices, and is green, gray, amber, or milky.

Notes

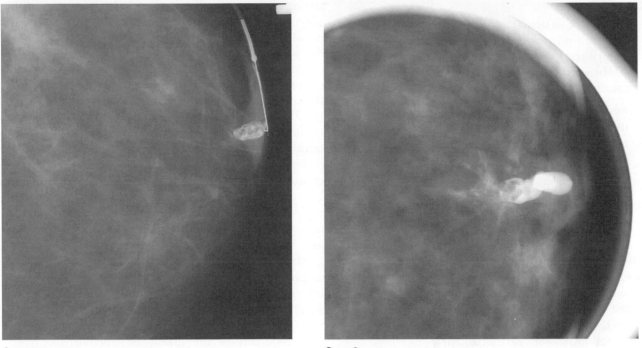

Case 1

Case 2

Shown are two examples of galactography.

1. What is the purpose of this study? What are the findings?

2. Are there any contraindications to performing galactography?

3. Describe the type and size of the cannula used and the contrast instilled during this procedure.

4. What other modalities may be used to evaluate patients with spontaneous nipple discharge?

Galactogram

1. The purpose of galactography or ductography is to determine the presence and location of intraductal lesions in patients with spontaneous nipple discharge. Both of these patients have intraductal masses that obstruct the ducts.

2. The only true contraindications are mastitis and a significant history of severe allergy to iodinated contrast.

3. Generally a blunt-tipped 30-gauge sialogram-type cannula is used with water-soluble contrast.

4. MRI and ultrasound have been used to evaluate patients with spontaneous nipple discharge.

References

Cardenosa G, Doudna C, Eklund GW: Ductography of the breast: Technique and findings, *Am J Roentgenol* 162:1081–1087, 1994.

Slawson SH, Johnson BA: Ductography: How to and what if? *RadioGraphics* 21:133, 2001.

Orel SG, Dougherty CS, Reynolds C, et al.: MR imaging in patients with nipple discharge: Initial experience, *Radiology* 216:248–254, 2000.

Cross-Reference

Ikeda, *Breast Imaging: THE REQUISITES*, p 292.

Comment

The steps in evaluating patients with spontaneous nipple discharge are controversial. First, the type of discharge and its true spontaneous nature must be determined. Many women are able to express discharge from their nipples on manipulation, but true spontaneous discharge is uncommon and requires a workup regardless of the nature of the discharge. If the discharge is bilateral and milky, hormonal levels (prolactin) are usually checked. However, if the discharge is bloody, clear, or serous and is from a single duct and truly spontaneous, further evaluation is necessary.

The purpose of a galactogram is to locate any intraductal lesions and map out the extent of the disease in the discharging duct. The procedure is generally simple. The discharging duct must be localized. Frequently, this requires a hot compress or heating pad to be placed on the nipple to relax the musculature of the nipple. Adequate lighting and magnification are often necessary to identify the opening of the duct. Often, the patient is able to demonstrate a trigger point in the breast that initiates the discharge. Once the discharging duct is localized, a 30-gauge blunt-tip sialogram cannula is gently placed into the duct orifice. The cannula is attached to tubing and a luerlock syringe filled with water-soluble contrast. The tubing must be checked carefully so that no air bubbles are present since bubbles injected into the ductal system may mimic intraductal lesions. The luerlock apparatus will help prevent additional air from entering the tubing system once it has been filled and the initial bubbles cleared. The contrast is instilled into the duct until the patient feels fullness in the breast or the contrast is seen spilling retrograde from the duct orifice. The procedure should not be painful. If the patient experiences any pain or burning when the contrast is injected, the injection should be stopped because the contrast may have extravasated outside of the ductal system into the surrounding parenchyma. Once a lesion or lesions have been mapped, the areas may be localized for surgical excision.

There is a wide spectrum of findings on galactography, but most significant are intraductal filling defects, obstruction, or wall irregularity or distortion. There is a significant overlap in the galactogram findings seen with papillomas and carcinomas. However, the greater the irregularity of the ductal architecture, the higher likelihood that there is a malignancy; any of these findings are suspicious and an excisional biopsy is recommended. Case 1 shows a lobulated distal intraductal mass that was shown to be a papilloma at excision. Case 2 was a small intraductal carcinoma.

Notes

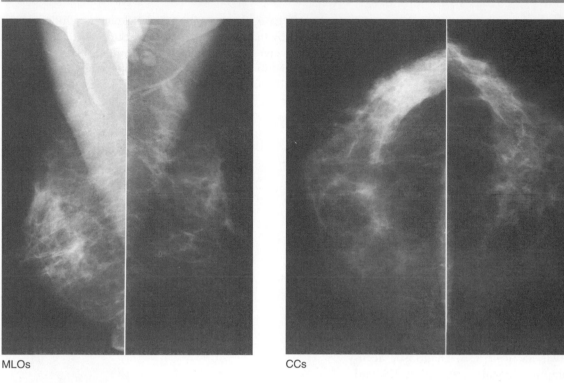

MLOs

CCs

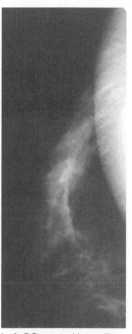

Left CC rotated laterally

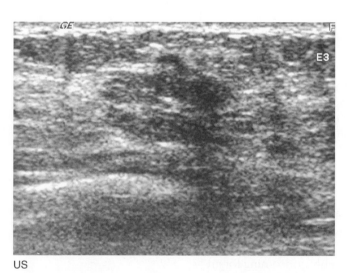

US

1. This 48-year-old woman presents with spontaneous left bloody nipple discharge. Describe the mammographic findings.

2. Describe the ultrasound findings of the lateral left breast.

3. What is the clinical concern?

4. What, if any, additional tests are recommended?

Bloody Nipple Discharge

1. The mammogram shows a focal asymmetry in the lateral left breast. This is best seen on the rotated cranial caudad view.

2. Ultrasound of the left breast at the 3 o'clock site shows a hypoechoic irregular mass that is suspicious for malignancy.

3. Because of the peripheral location of the ultrasound-detected mass, there is concern that there may be extension of disease along the ductal system toward the nipple causing the bloody nipple discharge.

4. A galactogram or MRI could be considered to better map out the extent of disease.

References

Berg WA, Gilbreath PL: Multicentric and multifocal cancer: Whole-breast US in preoperative evaluation, *Radiology* 214:59–66, 2000.

Berg WA, Gutierrez L, Ness Aiver MS, Carter WB, Bhargavan M, Lewis RS, Ioffe OB: Diagnostic accuracy of mammography, clinical examination, US, and MR imaging in preoperative assessment of breast cancer, *Radiology* 233:830–849, 2004.

Cross-Reference

Ikeda, *Breast Imaging: THE REQUISITES*, pp 292–294.

Comment

This patient presents with bloody nipple discharge and a subtle mammographic finding. The focal asymmetry in the lateral left breast is best seen on the rotated cranial caudad view. Although there is no definite distortion, calcifications, or suspicious mass, the patient was closely examined and the "trigger point" for her left nipple discharge was found along the 3 o'clock radius of the left breast, the same radius where the focal asymmetry is seen mammographically. Ultrasound was performed from the retroareolar area to the periphery of the breast at the 3 o'clock site, where the focal asymmetry is seen mammographically. A hypoechoic irregular mass with associated shadowing was found that corresponds in size and location to the mammographic lesion. The ultrasound finding is highly concerning for an area of invasive ductal carcinoma or a large focal mass of DCIS. Because of the history of bloody nipple discharge, there is concern for extension of disease toward the nipple from the peripherally located ultrasound finding. To further map out the extent of disease, an MRI or galactogram could be performed.

Preoperative ductography or MRI are recommended because blind surgical duct excision usually eliminates the discharge but may not actually reach the causative lesion.

In this case, the extent of disease was not fully appreciated by mammography or ultrasound, but on excision there were small foci of DCIS along the 3 o'clock radial duct distribution. This patient underwent mastectomy and had multifocal disease in the lateral left breast.

Notes

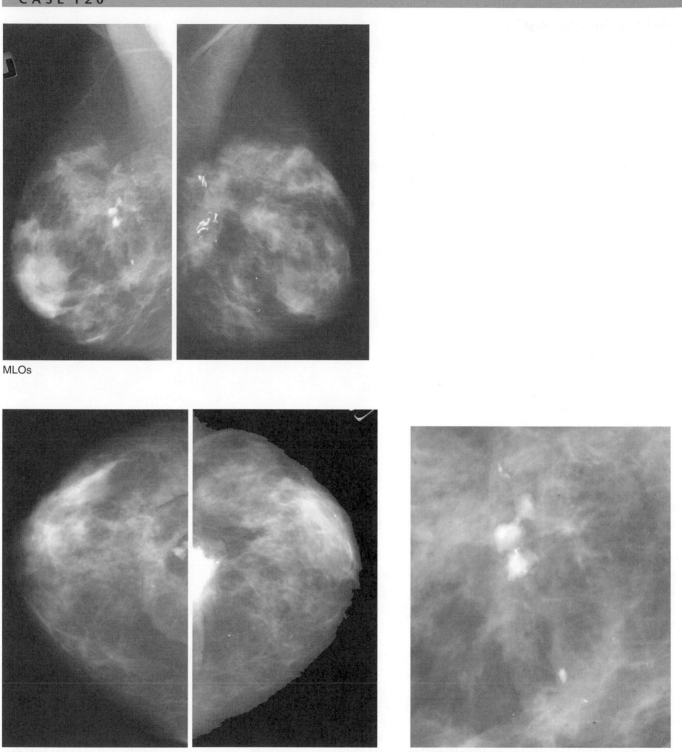

MLOs

CCs

Mag of left MLO

1. This 50-year-old woman presents for a screening mammogram. Describe the bilateral findings.

2. What is the most likely cause of the bilateral changes?

3. What is the high-density material due to? What are the calcifications from? In what location was the prior bilateral surgery?

4. What are the BI-RADS category and recommendation?

Post-Implant Removal

1. There are bilateral areas of high-density material associated with coarse dystrophic calcifications. There is a suggestion of slight architectural distortion in the posterior central breasts bilaterally. This is more pronounced on the cranial caudad views; however, the MLO views shows that no definite mass is seen.

2. This patient had bilateral silicone implants, which have been removed.

3. The high-density but noncalcific material seen in the left breast represents remaining free silicone in the breast tissue. The dystrophic calcifications are the residua of either capsular calcifications or fat necrosis following the removal of the bilateral silicone implants. The previous implants were in the retromammary or prepectoral location since the scarring is seen in front of the muscle.

4. After careful evaluation, there is no evidence of malignancy, but the report should describe the postsurgical changes and residual silicone in the breasts. BI-RADS category 2: benign, is appropriate.

Reference

Stewart NR, Monsees BS, Destouet JM, Rudloff MA: Mammographic appearance following implant removal, *Radiology* 185:83–85, 1992.

Cross-Reference

Ikeda, *Breast Imaging: THE REQUISITES*, p 262.

Comment

Initially, the cranial caudad views suggest bilateral spiculated masses or areas of architectural distortion. However, correlation of the cranial caudad views to the MLO views suggests that possible spiculation or distortion is actually superimposition due to the scarring from surgical procedures. The bilaterality, the presence of the dystrophic calcifications, and the small areas of high-density material are pathognemonic for the changes following explantation of bilaterally ruptured silicone implants. The high-density material is free silicone that is remaining in the breast tissue. This patient must be evaluated carefully to ensure that there are no signs of malignancy. The surgical changes may make this difficult, and magnification views and additional projections may be needed.

The location of the high-density material and scarring suggest that the implants were in the retromammary or prepectoral location and were silicone. A description of the findings should be included in the mammographic report for comparison with the patient's breast exam.

However, since there are no changes of malignancy and these are considered benign changes, a BI-RADS category 2 is adequate.

Notes

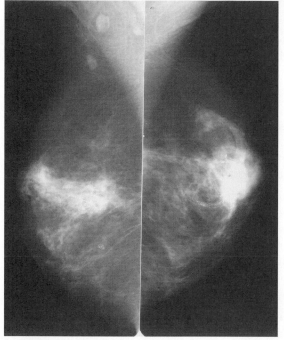

MLOs

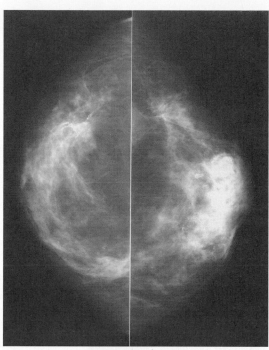

CCs

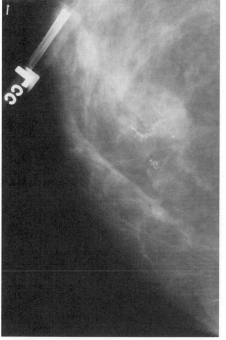

Mag view of left CC

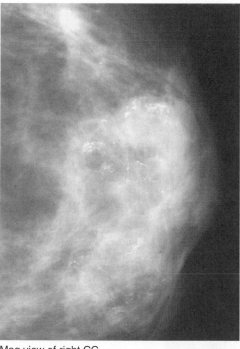

Mag view of right CC

1. This 45-year-old woman presents for a screening mammogram. What is the most likely pertinent history in this patient?

2. What characteristic mammographic findings are seen to support the history?

3. What are the calcifications from?

4. What BI-RADS category and assessment should be given?

Reduction

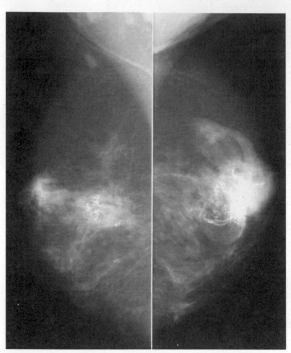

MLOs, 1 year later

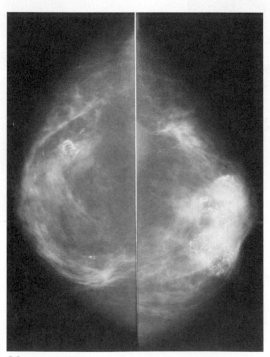

CCs, 1 year later

1. The patient has had a bilateral reduction mammoplasty.

2. There is displacement inferiorly of breast tissue, architectural distortion associated with surgical lines, and retroareolar fibrotic bands.

3. The calcifications are heterogeneous and follow along the surgical lines. The appearance is most consistent with early fat necrosis. If there is concern regarding the calcifications, a short-term follow-up to closely monitor the calcifications could be performed.

4. BI-RADS category 3, short-term follow-up recommended, is reasonable to ensure that the calcifications continue to mature as benign-appearing changes from the surgery; otherwise, a category 2, benign findings, when the calcifications are typical of the postsurgical changes.

Reference

Miller CL, Feig SA, Fox JW: Mammographic changes after reduction mammoplasty, *Am J Roentgenol* 149:35–38, 1987.

Cross-Reference

Ikeda, *Breast Imaging: THE REQUISITES*, p 271.

Comment

The patient has undergone bilateral reduction mammoplasty and the case demonstrates quite a few of the characteristic findings following this surgical procedure. The MLO views show that there is a somewhat wider contour than anterior projection of the breast. This is due to the removal of breast tissue inferiorly and the reduction of breast size, particularly in the anterior posterior direction. There is also the characteristic shift of the glandular tissue from the upper outer quadrant to a more inferior location. This is due to the surgical procedure, which removes tissue predominantly from the inferior breast. Extensive architectural distortion and fibrotic banding are seen along the surgical sutural lines. The calcifications are heterogeneous but are due to early fat necrosis. In the 1-year follow-up mammogram, the appearance of the calcifications has become more typical and the classic spherical lucencies of fat necrosis are also seen surrounded by the coarsening benign appearing calcifications. Of course, if there is clinical concern or suspicious mammographic findings, a biopsy must be recommended since cancer detection may be more difficult due to the postsurgical changes.

Notes

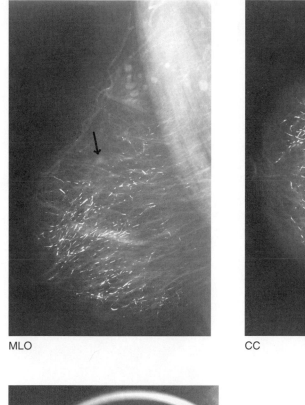

MLO

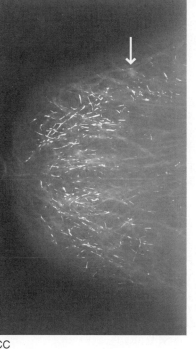

CC

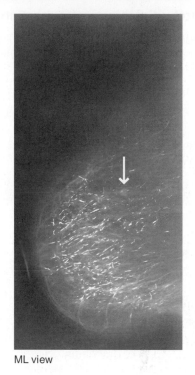

ML view

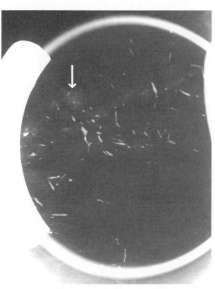

Spot mag CC

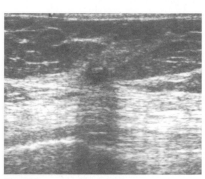

Rad US

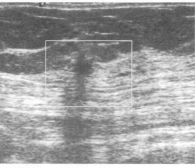

Arad US

1. Describe the findings on this left screening mammogram. What are the calcifications due to?

2. What other finding is present on the spot view?

3. Triangulate from the mammographic views and try to determine at what o'clock one would one look with ultrasound for this lesion.

4. Describe the ultrasound findings. What BI-RADS category should be given?

Secretory Calcifications with Cancer

1. There are diffuse calcifications consistent with secretory changes or plasma cell mastitis. The calcifications are benign.

2. There is a small irregular mass seen on the spot magnification view.

3. The mass is in the upper outer left breast, and a directed ultrasound, targeting the 2 o'clock site, was performed.

4. The small hypoechoic shadowing solid mass with irregular margins. BI-RADS category 4: suspicious, biopsy recommended.

Cross-Reference
Ikeda, *Breast Imaging: THE REQUISITES*, pp 41, 77.

Comment
On first glance, the calcifications in the left breast are quite impressive. This actually was a bilaterally symmetric process, and the branching, elongated, coarse calcifications are consistent with benign secretory changes. However, there is a small irregular mass in the upper outer aspect of the left breast. Triangulation suggests that this mass should be at approximately the 2 o'clock radii. A focused ultrasound was performed, and a small irregular mass was seen. The mass has some posterior acoustic shadowing and is taller than wide. The appearance is suspicious, and a BI-RADS category 4: suspicious, biopsy is recommended, was given. On ultrasound-guided core biopsy, this represented an invasive ductal carcinoma. This case illustrates the phenomena of "satisfaction of search." The calcifications are extensive, but diligence is necessary to exclude other subtle findings.

Notes

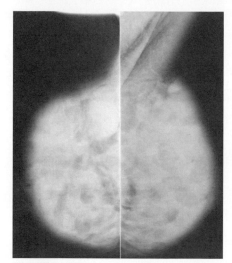

MLOs, case 1

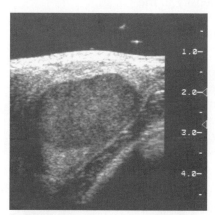

Radial US, case 1

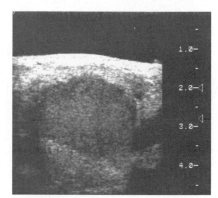

Antiradial US, case 1

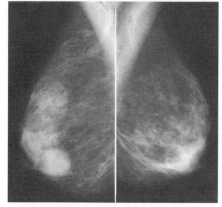

MLOs, case 2

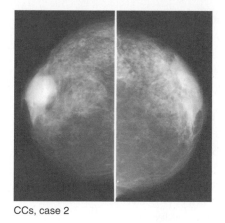

CCs, case 2

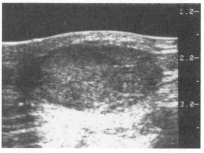

Radial US, case 2

1. Case 1 is a 35-year-old with a new palpable left breast mass. Case 2 is a 72-year-old with a new palpable breast mass. Describe the mammographic features of each.

2. Describe the ultrasound features of each. How important is the presence of posterior acoustic enhancement in the differential diagnosis?

3. What is the most likely diagnosis for the 35-year-old and for the 72-year-old?

4. How common are circumscribed breast cancers?

Circumscribed Breast Cancer

1. Each patient presents with a mass seen on the mammogram. Because of the high density in the young woman, the mass is not well differentiated from the surrounding dense glandular tissue, but is partially seen in the left axillary tail.

2. The ultrasounds of both patients show a homogeneous solid mass with posterior acoustic enhancement. Posterior acoustic enhancement may be seen in either benign or malignant lesions. Careful inspection of the borders of these masses shows that there is not a thin echogenic margin but, rather, a poorly defined or irregular margin.

3. The most likely diagnosis for the 35-year-old is a benign fibroadenoma despite the slightly irregular margin. However, for the 72-year-old, the most likely diagnosis for a new solid mass is invasive ductal carcinoma. Both of these lesions proved malignant.

4. Circumscribed breast cancers present less than 10% of the time.

Reference

Stavros TA: *Breast Ultrasound*, Philadelphia, 2004, Lippincott Williams & Wilkins.

Cross-Reference

Ikeda, *Breast Imaging: THE REQUISITES*, pp 105–108.

Comment

This case demonstrates circumscribed cancers in two patients, one relatively young and the other older. The differential diagnosis is different for the two patients because of the incidence of breast cancer in their respective age groups. In the younger woman, a fibroadenoma would be a more likely diagnosis for this solid mass. However, on careful inspection, the ultrasound shows that portions of the mass margins are irregular, and therefore the mass is suspicious. In the older postmenopausal patient, a new solid mass must be considered cancer until proven otherwise.

There is posterior acoustic enhancement seen in both of these malignant cases. Although this is often considered a sign of benignity, malignant masses may also demonstrate posterior acoustic enhancement. The degree of enhancement depends on the homogeneity of the internal aspect of the mass. In both cases, the internal cellular contents of the malignant masses are very homogeneous and the malignant masses demonstrate posterior acoustic enhancement. Core biopsy was performed on both of these masses, and both were invasive ductal carcinomas, not otherwise specified.

Notes

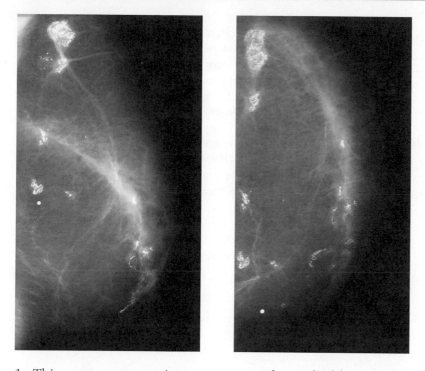

1. This mastectomy patient presents with a palpable mass in the upper outer quadrant of the transverse rectus abdominus musculocutaneous (TRAM) flap reconstruction. What is your interpretation of the diagnostic mammogram?

2. Is this patient at an increased risk of breast cancer?

3. What is the imaging evaluation for a palpable lump in the reconstructed breast?

4. Is any additional evaluation needed for this patient?

Palpable Mass in TRAM

1. The mammogram shows a TRAM reconstruction with several groups of coarse calcifications. In the upper outer quadrant, the calcifications are clumped into mass-like areas. This is characteristic of fat necrosis.

2. The breast cancer survivor is at an increased risk of developing additional breast cancer. Palpable masses must be thoroughly evaluated.

3. As in the native breast, the evaluation begins with mammography. Ultrasound and MRI can be used for further characterization of a palpable finding if the mammogram is not diagnostic.

4. In this patient, the palpable finding corresponds to an area of fat lucency with associated coarse calcifications, characteristic of fat necrosis. No further evaluation is necessary.

References

Eidelman Y, Liebling RW, Buchbinder S, Strauch B, Goldstein RD: Mammography in the evaluation of masses in breasts reconstructed with TRAM flaps, *Ann Plast Surg* 41(3):229–233, 1998.

Helvie MA, Bailey JE, Roubidoux MA, Pass HA, Chang AE, Pierce LJ, Wilkins EG: Mammographic screening of TRAM flap breast reconstructions for detection of nonpalpable recurrent cancer, *Radiology* 224:211, 2002.

Pang LM, Chan E, Yang WT: Florid dystrophic calcification associated with fatty degeneration of muscle component in the TRAM flap, *Am J Roentgenol* 177:1489, 2001.

Cross-Reference

Ikeda, *Breast Imaging: THE REQUISITES*, p 271.

Comment

One common method of breast reconstruction after mastectomy is the TRAM flap. Skin, fat, and rectus muscle are brought up from the abdomen to construct a breast mound. This procedure uses living tissue from the mastectomy patient (autogenous transplant).

Fat necrosis after a surgical procedure is not uncommon because areas of fat can lose their blood supply during the procedure. The area of fatty tissue death can calcify, and the calcifications may initially appear as pleomorphic shapes that, in time, become coarse, often with associated fat lucency.

The mechanism of malignancy developing in the TRAM is not entirely understood, but possibilities include residual cancer tissue, tumor seeding at the time of mastectomy, and tumor sequestered in lymphatics. It may also develop in remnants of native breast tissue not removed entirely at mastectomy.

Differentiating fat necrosis calcifications from malignant calcifications can be difficult. The patient who has undergone a mastectomy for malignant disease is at increased risk to develop a new breast cancer or a recurrence of the known cancer.

The patient in this example presented with a palpable finding, and a diagnostic mammogram was performed of the TRAM flap. Although it is controversial, it may be useful to perform routine screening mammography of the TRAM reconstruction at the time of the mammogram of the remaining breast. Helvie and colleagues noted that malignancy was found as nonpalpable lesions in the TRAM flap in 2% of cases, approximately the same rate of malignancy found after breast conservation therapy.

Notes

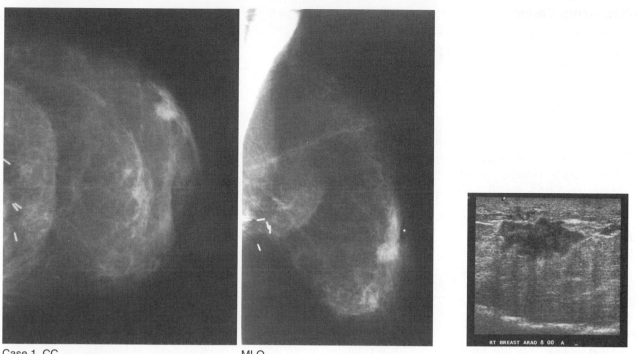

Case 1, CC   MLO

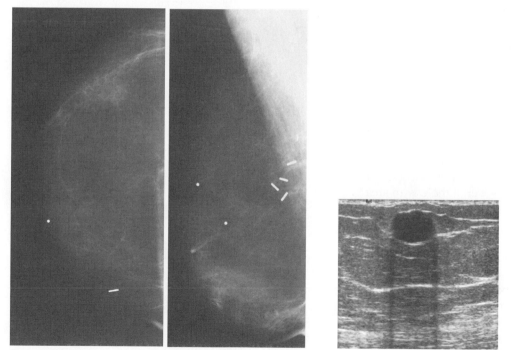

Case 2, CC   MLO

1. The images are of two patients who have had the same procedure. What is the surgical procedure?

2. Both patients have areas of palpable concern and BBs were placed over the site of concern. Describe the mammographic findings in both cases.

3. Describe the ultrasound findings of both patients.

4. What is the most likely diagnosis in each case?

TRAM Flap—Two Cases

1. The patients have both had transverse rectus abdominus myocutaneous (TRAM) flaps following skin-sparing mastectomies.

2. In case 1, mammography reveals an irregular mass at the site of palpable concern. In case 2, there is a lucent, well-circumscribed mass.

3. In case 1, ultrasound reveals an irregular solid mass with overlying skin thickening. In case 2, there is a well-defined hypo- to anechoic mass

4. Case 1: cancer recurrence. Case 2: fat necrosis.

Reference

Helvie MA, Wilson TE, Roubidoux MA, Wilkins EG, Chang AE: Mammographic appearance of recurrent breast carcinoma in six patients with TRAM flap breast reconstructions, *Radiology* 209:711–715, 1998.

Cross-Reference

Ikeda, *Breast Imaging: THE REQUISITES*, pp 270–271.

Comment

These patients underwent skin-sparing mastectomies with immediate TRAM flap reconstruction. The MLO and CC views of both patients show the typical surgical changes of the rectus abdominus muscle transposed with the fatty abdominal subcutaneous tissue. The adipose tissue from the abdomen makes up the bulk of the breast mound, and the clips posteriorly secure the transposed rectus muscle to the chest wall. In these cases, the nipple and areola have been removed, but the remainder of the original breast skin was maintained, hence the term skin-sparing mastectomy. Routine mammographic imaging of the TRAM flap is controversial; however, if there is an area of concern on exam, directed imaging is always necessary.

In case 1, the irregular mass seen mammographically and also on ultrasound is due to a recurrence of the patient's cancer along a scar line. The mammographic and ultrasound appearance of cancer recurrence in a TRAM flap is similar to that of a primary breast carcinoma. The mass in poorly defined on mammography and is irregular and hypoechoic on ultrasound. The patient underwent ultrasound core biopsy and a recurrence was confirmed.

In case 2, the diagnosis of fat necrosis can be made based on the mammographic appearance at the site of the TRAM flap, but the ultrasound also confirms the diagnosis. In this case, no further evaluation is needed and the patient may be reassured that the clinical findings are due to postoperative changes only.

Notes

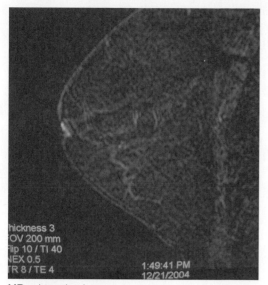

hickness 3
OV 200 mm
lip 10 / TI 40
NEX 0.5
TR 8 / TE 4   1:49:41 PM
                          12/21/2004

MR subtraction image

1. This patient's physician noted a unilateral inverted nipple on routine exam. The patient was unaware of the abnormality. Her mammogram is normal except for the inverted nipple. What is your interpretation of the subtraction MR image?

2. What is the concern in a patient with an inverted nipple?

3. What is the workup for inverted nipple?

4. What follow-up is indicated after the MRI?

MRI of Inverted Nipple

1. There is minimal enhancement of the nipple, which is inverted. There is no evidence of enhancing mass.

2. A retroareolar malignancy can cause the nipple to invert.

3. A history should be obtained. Standard mammographic views and spot compression views of the nipple should be performed. Ultrasound may be useful to evaluate the retroareolar area.

4. The patient can be recommended to return for routine screening and clinical follow-up.

Reference

Friedman EP, Hall-Craggs MA, Mumtaz H, Schneidau A: Breast MR and the appearance of the normal and abnormal nipple, *Clin Radiol* 52(11):854–861, 1997.

Cross-Reference

Ikeda, *Breast Imaging: THE REQUISITES*, pp 26, 34.

Comment

If routine imaging (mammography and ultrasound) are normal, MRI is a useful next step in a situation where there is an unexplained clinical finding. This patient was seen on routine clinical exam to have an inverted nipple. A mammogram, which was negative, showed a fatty breast. No mass that would explain the nipple inversion was noted. The referring physician then requested an MRI.

In the setting of an inverted nipple, it is important to obtain a clinical history. Has the nipple been inverted for many years? An acutely inverted nipple is of concern for malignancy, and a chronically inverted nipple is not.

If the nipple inversion is chronic, no additional workup is required. This is a common benign condition and may be caused by periductal fibrosis and chronic duct ectasia. An acutely inverted nipple is a new clinical finding and may represent a sign of malignancy. A retroareolar mass can cause the nipple to invert, just as a mass in the peripheral breast can cause skin retraction and dimpling. The workup for acute nipple inversion includes a mammogram, which should include spot compression views of the retroareolar area. This area of the breast has many overlapping normal structures, and a small mass may be present and not seen on the standard views. If no mass is seen on mammography, ultrasound is a valuable exam. If no mass is seen on ultrasound in the setting of an acutely inverted nipple, MRI is recommended.

On MRI, evaluate the images for an enhancing mass or ductal enhancement in the retroareolar breast. Ductal enhancement can indicate DCIS. The nipple itself will commonly enhance on MRI. In this patient, the MRI shows normal minimal enhancement of the nipple and no evidence of an enhancing mass. No further imaging work up is necessary.

Notes

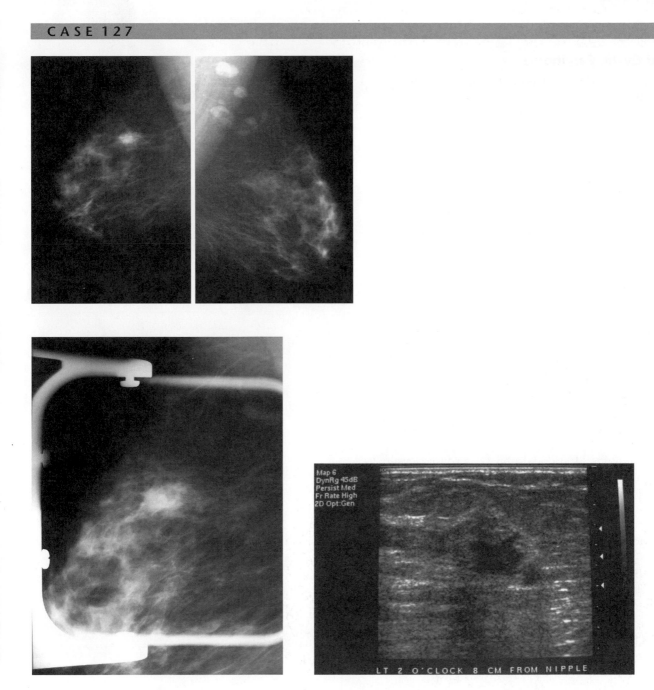

1. Describe the mammogram and ultrasound findings.

2. What is the most common subtype of breast cancer?

3. Why is it useful to know the pathologic subtype of a breast cancer?

4. What are the rare types of invasive breast cancer?

Adenoid Cystic Carcinoma

1. There is a high-density mass in the upper outer left breast with microlobulated margins that persists on spot compression view and also a hypoechoic, irregular mass with posterior shadowing on ultrasound.

2. Invasive ductal cancer is the most common. The NOS (not otherwise specified) subtype represents 70–80% of all breast cancers.

3. The pathologic subtype often predicts the prognosis of the cancer.

4. Adenoid cystic carcinoma, secretory carcinoma, squamous cell carcinoma, and metaplastic carcinoma are rare subtypes of breast cancer.

References

Arpino G, Clark GM, Mohsin S, Bardou VJ, Elledge RM: Adenoid cystic carcinoma of the breast: Molecular markers, treatment, and clinical outcome, *Cancer* 94(8):2119–2127, 2002.

Bourke AG, Metcalf C, Wylie EJ: Mammographic features of adenoid cystic carcinoma, *Aust Radiol* 38(4):324–325, 1994.

Leeming R, Jenkins M, Mendelsohn G: Adenoid cystic carcinoma of the breast, *Arch Surg* 127(2):233–235, 1992.

Santamaría G, Velasco M, Zanón G: Adenoid cystic carcinoma of the breast: Mammographic appearance and pathologic correlation, *Am J Roentgenol* 171:1679, 1998.

Sperber F, Blank A, Metser U: Adenoid cystic carcinoma of the breast: Mammographic, sonographic, and pathological correlation, *Breast J* 8(1):53–54, 2002.

Cross-Reference

Ikeda, *Breast Imaging: THE REQUISITES*, p 116.

Comment

There are unusual cell types of breast cancer including adenoid cystic carcinoma, which represents less than 1% of all breast cancers. This subtype rarely spreads beyond the breast to the lymph nodes or to distant sites. Its appearance on mammography and ultrasound is similar to other breast cancers, most often presenting as a lobulated mass.

It is important to know the cell type of breast cancers because the cell type often determines the clinical outcome. Adenoid cystic carcinoma has a better prognosis than other types. In a study of 28 patients with adenoid cystic carcinoma, the 5-year disease-free survival was 100%. This excellent prognosis affects treatment options: Axillary dissection is not necessary, nor is chemotherapy. However, the mass must be completely excised or recurrence may occur in the breast. The average age of diagnosis is postmenopausal, age 65 years.

In our patient, a developing irregular high-density mass with microlobulated margins was seen in the upper outer quadrant of the left breast on routine screening mammogram. She was 63 years old when diagnosed, and on pathology a 2-cm mass was predominantly *in situ* adenoid cystic cancer, with rare areas of invasion.

Notes

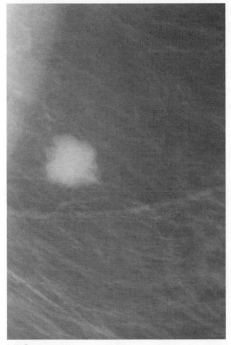

MLO mag

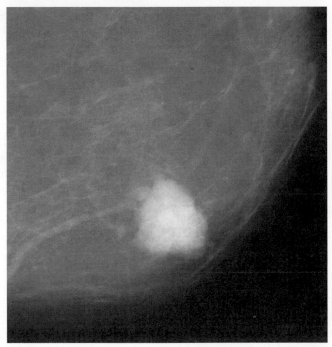

CC mag

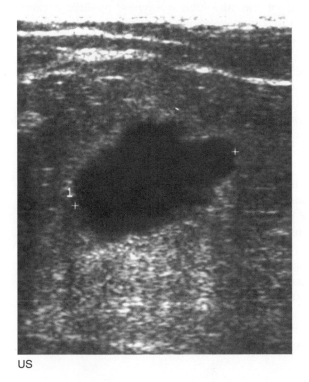

US

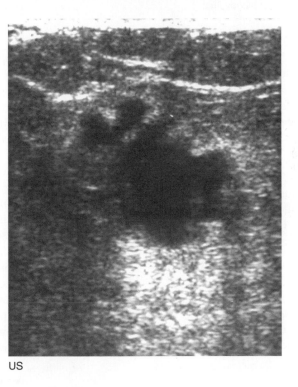

US

1. Describe the mammographic findings in this 45-year-old woman.

2. Describe the ultrasound findings and give a BI-RADS category and recommendation.

3. An aspiration was performed and the mass decreased significantly in size, but the aspirated material was grossly bloody. What is the next recommendation?

4. What type of cancer often presents as a circumscribed mass?

Medullary Cancer

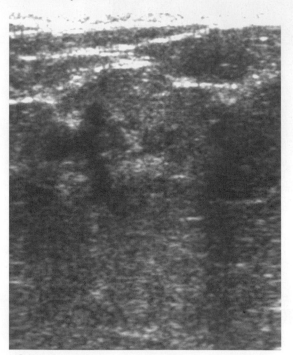

US following aspiraton of bloody fluid

1. There is a microlobulated, well-defined mass in the right breast.

2. Ultrasound demonstrates a very hypoechoic to anechoic microlobulated mass that has thick walls. BI-RADS 4: suspicious, biopsy is recommended. The radiologist thought that this might be a complex cyst and an aspiration was performed.

3. Although the mass decreased significantly in size, the finding of a bloody aspirate is concerning. Careful evaluation of the postaspiration ultrasound image reveals that a small irregular hypoechoic mass remains. Excisional biopsy or a core biopsy of the residual mass is necessary.

4. The most common cancer that presents as a circumscribed mass is an invasive ductal carcinoma, not otherwise specified (NOS). However, of the histologic subtypes frequently circumscribed, medullary is one of the most common. This case is an example of a necrotic medullary carcinoma.

References

Bassett LW, Jackson VP, Jahan R, Fu YS, Gold RH: *Diagnosis of Diseases of the Breast*, Philadelphia, 1997, Saunders.

Berg WA, Campassi CI, Ioffe OB: Cystic lesions of the breast: Sonographic–pathologic correlation, *Radiology* 227:183, 2003.

Cross-Reference

Ikeda, *Breast Imaging: THE REQUISITES*, p 146.

Comment

This microlobulated mass seen on mammography has fairly well-circumscribed margins. The ultrasound shows that there are thick irregular walls that are suspicious for this being more than just a complex cyst. The mass looks very hypoechoic, almost anechoic, and this degree of microlobulation is rarely seen in benign cysts. An aspiration was performed and the mass almost entirely disappeared. However, the aspirate was grossly bloody and was sent to cytology. Although the mass decreased significantly in size, as shown in the image, the grossly bloody aspirate was highly concerning for aspiration of a necrotic tumor and excision was recommended. (An alternative to excision would have been to perform a core biopsy under ultrasound at the time of the aspiration.) A necrotic medullary carcinoma was found at excision.

Medullary carcinomas are often called circumscribed cancers. The most common cancer to present as a circumscribed mass is an invasive ductal carcinoma, NOS. However, of the histologic subtypes, medullary carcinoma most often presents as a circumscribed mass. Medullary carcinoma presents in a slightly younger age group (younger than 50 years) than invasive ductal carcinoma, NOS, but it accounts for less than 10% of breast cancers. Mammographically, calcifications are unusual in this subtype of invasive ductal carcinoma.

Ultrasound frequently demonstrates round or lobulated hypoechoic masses due to the central necrosis of the tumor. In this case, careful analysis of the margins reveals microlobulation, thick walls, and irregularity. These tumors often exhibit posterior acoustic enhancement due to the homogeneity of the internal cellular structures or because of internal tumor necrosis. Histologically, these tumors have a prominent lymphoplasmocytic infiltration and have large pleomorphic nuclei with prominent nucleoli and high mitotic activity. They have a fast rate of growth, larger size at presentation, and more often have negative hormonal markers compared to invasive ductal carcinoma, NOS. Despite the rapid growth rate, they tend to have a slightly better prognosis than invasive ductal carcinoma, NOS.

Notes

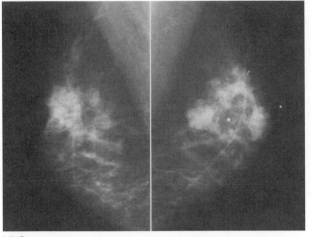

MLOs

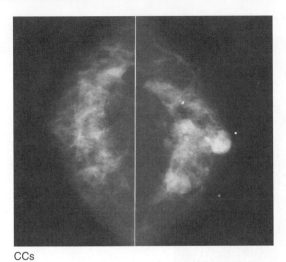

CCs

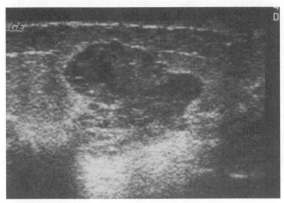

Right US at 12:00

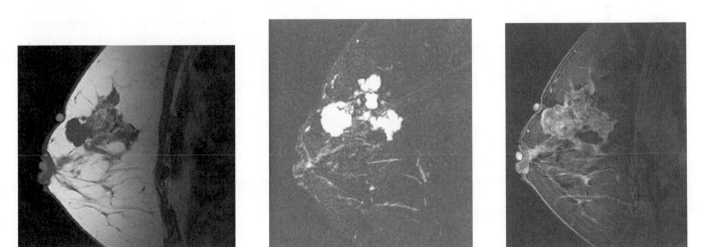

Right MRI, T1

T2

Post Gd

1. This 72-year-old woman presents with palpable masses at 12:00 in the right breast. Describe the mammographic findings.

2. Describe the ultrasound finding.

3. Describe the MRI findings.

4. What is the differential diagnosis?

Multifocal Mucinous Carcinoma

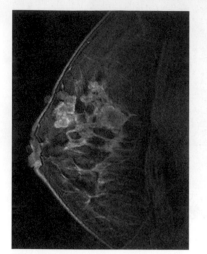

MR subtraction image

1. Mammographically, there are multiple high-density masses in the right breast. The margins of the masses are partially obscured.

2. On ultrasound, the masses have irregular margins and are isoechoic to fat. They do demonstrate posterior acoustic enhancement but are clearly not simple cysts. In addition, the margins of the masses are irregular.

3. The multiple masses have a very high signal on T2, suggesting that they are cystic or filled with a proteinaceous material. There is a progressive enhancement pattern, and the masses show minimal rim enhancement on delayed gadolinium imaging.

4. The differential diagnosis is mucinous carcinoma vs multiple inflamed complex cysts. FNA of the right breast masses demonstrated mucinous carcinoma.

References

Conant EF, Dillon RL, Palazzo J, Ehrlich SM, Feig SA: Imaging findings in mucin-containing carcinomas of the breast: Correlation with pathologic features, *Am J Roentgenol* 163:821–824, 1994.

Kawashima M, Tamaki Y, Nonaka Y, Higuchi K, Kimura M, Koida T, Yanagita, Y, Sugihara S: MR imaging of mucinous carcinoma of the breast, *Am J Roentgenol* 179:179–183, 2002.

Lam WWM, Chu WCW, Tse GM, Ma TK: Sonographic appearance of mucinous carcinoma of the breast, *Am J Roentgenol* 182:1069–1074, 2004.

Cross-Reference

Ikeda, *Breast Imaging: THE REQUISITES*, pp 106, 144, 206.

Comment

Mucinous carcinoma is a subtype of invasive ductal carcinoma that accounts for less than 5% of breast carcinomas. Mucinous carcinomas tend to occur in older women and a very slow growth rate, a low tendency to metastasize, and, therefore, a much better prognosis than invasive ductal carcinoma, not otherwise specified (NOS). Synonyms for mucinous carcinoma include colloid carcinoma and gelatinous carcinoma. These lesions may be screen detected in asymptomatic patients or may present as palpable, rubbery breast masses, which may be quite large.

On gross pathology, pure mucinous carcinomas tend to be gelatinous, and their macroscopic cut surfaces may glisten due to the high mucin content. Histologically, the tumor cells are seen floating within the abundant extracellular mucin. Tumors having less than 75% mucin component are classified as mixed cancers, and the prognosis is less favorable compared to that for the pure forms. The mixed forms tend to have a similar prognosis as that for invasive ductal carcinoma, NOS.

Mammographically, the masses are often round and well circumscribed or have partially fading or obscured margins. Calcifications are rarely seen in pure mucinous carcinoma; however, as the amount of NOS carcinoma increases in mixed forms, the appearance of the tumor tends to be more typical of invasive ductal carcinoma and calcifications and spiculation may be present. Ultrasonographically, the lesions are often fairly well defined but may have microlobulated margins and appear hypoechoic or isoechoic to the surrounding breast tissue. MRI may show a high signal on T2 due to the abundant proteinaceous mucin material. Enhancement is often minimal on MRI, as in this case, and care must be taken to not incorrectly diagnose these lesions on MRI as inflamed cyst. Subtraction images may be helpful to demonstrate the minimal enhancement at the periphery of the lesions.

Notes

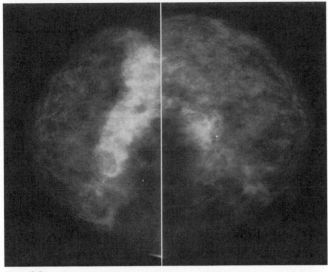

First CCs

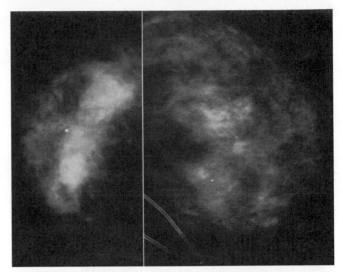

CCs 3 years later

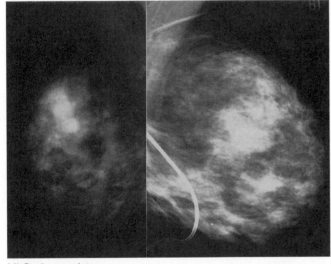

MLOs 3 years later

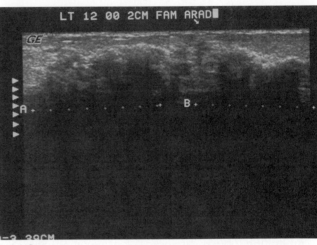

Left US

This 45-year-old woman presents with a complaint of a shrinking left breast. She is a long-standing insulin-dependent diabetic. Presented above are images 3 years apart.

1. Describe the mammographic findings.

2. Why is the breast shrinking?

3. What is the differential diagnosis?

4. What procedure would you recommend?

Invasive Lobular Carcinoma—Shrinking Breast

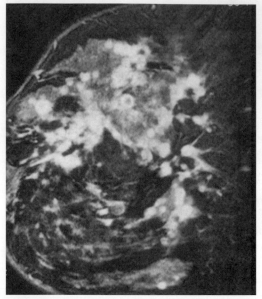

Left MRI

1. The mammographic finding falls under the descriptor "global asymmetry." However, of note is that the denser breast is also shrinking in size over time.

2. The shrinking is due to a diffuse process that is causing retraction of the normal breast parenchyma.

3. The leading diagnoses are diffuse involvement of diabetic mastopathy or invasive lobular carcinoma.

4. Either entity can be diagnosed by core biopsy.

References

Harvey JA, Fechner RE, Moore MM: Apparent ipsilateral decrease in breast size on mammography: A sign of infiltrating lobular carcinoma, *Radiology* 213:883–889, 2000.

Qayyum A, Birdwell RL, Daniel BL, Nowels KW, Jeffrey SS, Agoston TA, Herfkens RJ: MR imaging features of infiltrating lobular carcinoma of the breast: Histopathologic correlation, *Am J Roentgenol* 178(5):1227–1232, 2002.

Cross-Reference

Ikeda, *Breast Imaging: THE REQUISITES*, pp 97–98, 206, 236.

Comment

A decrease in breast size or a "shrinking breast" has been described when there is diffuse involvement of infiltrating lobular carcinoma (ILC) as in this case. Included in the differential diagnosis is diabetic mastopathy, which may also cause dense fibrosis and a decrease in the breast size. The ultrasound images show diffuse shadowing due to difficulty penetrating the band of desmoplastic tissue in the superior breast. MRI shows multiple rim enhancing nodules extending from the upper medial and lateral breast as well as some extension into the inferior breast. MRI better shows the extent of the tumor compared to either mammography or ultrasound. Core biopsy was performed under ultrasound guidance to diagnose the mammography.

ILC accounts for approximately 10% of breast cancers and is infamous for being difficult to diagnose mammographically. ILC most commonly presents mammographically as an area of focal asymmetry or subtle architectural distortion. The lesions may be difficult to diagnose because the single cells of the tumor infiltrate through the fat and stroma without causing much architectural change or mass effect. The tumors generally present at a larger size than invasive ductal carcinoma. Also, because of the frequent lack of discrete mammographic findings and the low density of the tumor, ILC is associated with a higher mammographic false-negative rate than infiltrating ductal carcinoma. ILC presents as multicentric disease, as in this case, twice as often as does invasive ductal carcinoma.

A decrease in breast size has been described with advanced cases of ILC as well as with focal involvement of the tumor. Patients may complain only of diffuse thickening of the breasts. Occasionally, patients present with focal areas of discrete masses or multiple areas of nodularity. In patients with decreasing breast size due to ILC, there may be extensive disease with numerous microscopic skip areas and multicentricity. Dense fibrotic tissue formation is due to the stromal response to the lobular tumor cells. MRI is helpful in establishing the extent of disease. This patient had multiple positive nodes and underwent mastectomy.

Notes

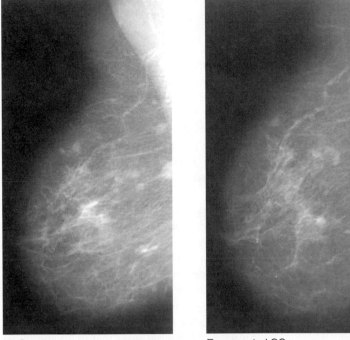

MLO

Exaggerated CC

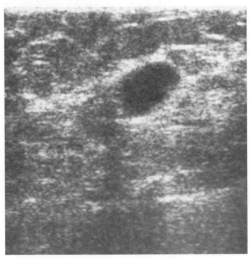

US

1. This 74-year-old woman presents with palpable left axillary adenopathy. Describe the findings seen on the left breast images.

2. Give a differential diagnosis for the mammographic and ultrasound findings.

3. The patient has a history of non-Hodgkin's lymphoma. Which is more common, primary lymphomatous involvement of the breast or metastatic involvement?

4. How does the appearance of primary lymphoma of the breast differ from metastatic lymphoma?

Lymphoma

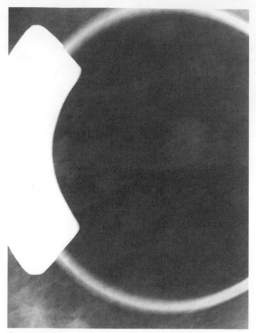

Spot mag

1. There are multiple masses in the left breast, many of which have obscured or fading margins.
The ultrasound shows an extremely hypoechoic mass that does not fulfill all the criteria of a simple cyst (no sharp, thin margin but, rather, a thick margin in portions). There were multiple similar-appearing masses in the left breast on ultrasound.

2. The differential diagnosis of these multiple masses includes lymphomatous involvement of the breast and multiple metastases from an extramammary primary.

3. Metastatic involvement from extramammary lymphoma is more common than primary lymphoma of the breast.

4. The appearance of primary lymphoma of the breast may be similar to that of metastases from extramammary lymphoma; however, the majority of primary lymphomas present as a solitary noncalcified mass. In this case, with the history of extramammary lymphoma and the presentation of multiple masses and lymphadenopathy, metastatic involvement of lymphoma is most likely.

Reference

Liberman L, Giess CS, Dershaw DD, et al.: Non-Hodgkin lymphoma of the breast: Imaging characteristics and correlation with histopathologic findings, *Radiology* 192:157–160, 1994.

Cross-Reference

Ikeda, *Breast Imaging: THE REQUISITES*, p 117.

Comment

The most likely diagnosis in this patient is breast involvement from her known extramammary non-Hodgkin's lymphoma. However, the multiple masses could easily be due to metastases from an unknown primary malignancy, such as lung carcinoma or melanoma.

The majority of primary lymphomas present as solitary noncalcified masses on mammography. The masses of either primary or metastatic lymphoma are usually noncalcified and have incompletely circumscribed or obscured margins, but 30% present as circumscribed masses. On ultrasound, the solid lymphoma nodules may be extremely hypoechoic and often have a pseudocystic appearance, as in this case. A core biopsy is recommended, rather than a FNA, so that flow cytometry studies may be performed to determine the type of lymphoma.

Primary lymphoma of the breast is rare and usually presents with a solitary palpable mass that may often have skin changes, such as retraction, erythema, or thickening. In primary lymphoma of the breast, axillary nodal involvement is common, with approximately 30–40% of cases presenting this way. Involvement of both breasts in primary lymphoma is found in 13% of cases. If the breast involvement from a primary lymphoma is small, treatment may be limited to breast conservation and radiation.

Notes

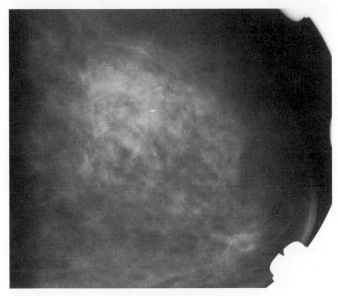

Magnification spot view of right breast

1. The calcifications in the right breast were sampled with stereotactic biopsy. Pathology showed several foci of lobular carcinoma *in situ* (LCIS) and benign calcifications associated with fibrocystic change. Does this patient need surgery?

2. Is this patient at increased risk of breast cancer?

3. Is the risk of developing cancer at the site of the LCIS?

4. Is there increased risk for developing ductal or lobular cancer?

Management of LCIS

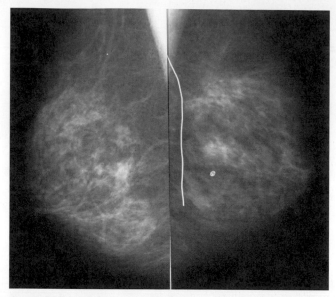

Cropped MLO views 1 year later with scar marker on right

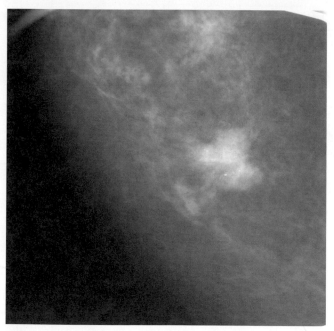

Left spot mag 1 year later

1. Surgery is recommended, but the LCIS was an incidental finding not associated with the mammographically suspicious calcifications. The mammographic abnormality was benign on pathology.

2. Yes, she has an approximately 27–30% increased risk of developing breast cancer.

3. The increased risk of developing cancer applies to both breasts.

4. The risk of developing cancer is for both ductal and lobular cancers.

References

Berg WA, Mrose HE, and Ioffe OB: Atypical lobular hyperplasia or lobular carcinoma in situ at core-needle breast biopsy, *Radiology* 218:503–509, 2001.

Foster MC, Helvie MA, Gregory NE, Rebner M, Nees AV, Paramagul C: Lobular carcinoma in situ or atypical lobular hyperplasia at core-needle biopsy: Is excisional biopsy necessary? *Radiology* 231(3):813–819, 2004.

Liberman L, Sama M, Susnik B, et al.: Lobular carcinoma in situ at percutaneous breast biopsy: Surgical biopsy findings, *Am J Roentgenol* 173:291–299, 1999.

Cross-Reference

Ikeda, *Breast Imaging: THE REQUISITES*, pp 25, 184.

Comment

LCIS is a high-risk lesion and an important risk factor for future development of breast cancer. The increased risk is for both breasts, not specifically at the site where the LCIS was found. In this patient, microcalcifications present in the right breast were biopsied and shown to be fibrocystic changes with multiple foci of LCIS. The LCIS was not associated with the calcifications and was an incidental finding, as is often the case. The following year, a new mass with associated calcifications was seen in the contralateral breast. It was sampled with the core needle technique and shown to be invasive ductal cancer.

Patients with LCIS are at approximately 27–30% increased risk for developing breast cancer. LCIS is detected on image-guided biopsy and at excisional biopsy for calcifications and masses, and it is usually an incidental finding. It has no imaging features of its own. The risk of subsequent cancer increases when multiple lobules of LCIS are seen on histopathology. The pathology of the future cancer can be either ductal or lobular.

Excisional biopsy is recommended in patients who have LCIS at core needle biopsy because there is a 10–20% chance that there is DCIS or invasive cancer near the site of LCIS at core needle biopsy and the core sampling did not represent the entire lesion. The same is true for core biopsies showing atypical lobular hyperplasia and atypical ductal hyperplasia.

Notes

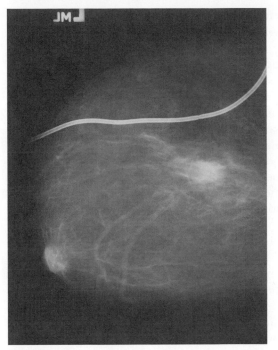

ML view

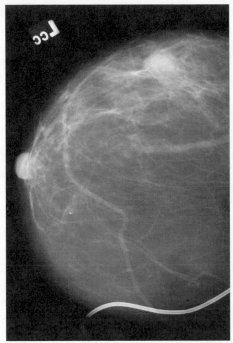

CC view

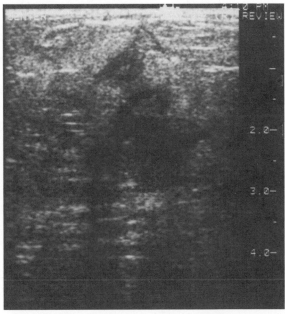

US

1. Describe the mammographic findings in this 36-year-old woman with a tender palpable left breast mass.

2. What clinical questions of the patient might be helpful in determining the etiology of this abnormality? What is the radiopaque line seen along the upper inner aspect of the breast?

3. Describe the ultrasound findings and give a differential diagnosis.

4. Assign a BI-RADS category and discuss the management of this lesion.

Abscess

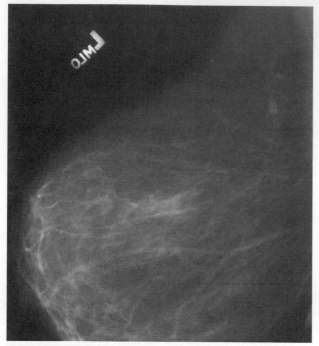

Follow-up mammo 4 weeks later

1. There is a poorly defined mass in the upper outer quadrant of the left breast.

2. The patient should be asked about how long the area has been palpable and tender. If there are any skin changes, the technologist should note them on the patient questionnaire. The line is an indwelling catheter.

3. On ultrasound, there is a poorly defined hypoechoic area that is taller than wide and extends toward the skin surface; there is surrounding edema. The differential diagnosis includes cancer, an abscess, and a hematoma.

4. If there are clinical changes that suggest an infection, the patient could be treated with antibiotics and followed (BI-RADS 3). If there are no clinical findings consistent with an abscess, a biopsy is necessary (BI-RADS 4).

References

Berg WA, Campassi CI, Ioffe OB: Cystic lesions of the breast: Sonographic–pathologic correlation, *Radiology* 227:183, 2003.

Ulitzsch D, Nyman MKG, Carlson RA: Breast abscess in lactating women: US-guided treatment, *Radiology* 232:904–909, 2004.

Cross-Reference

Ikeda, *Breast Imaging: THE REQUISITES*, pp 126–128.

Comment

The mammogram shows a poorly defined mass in the lateral breast that corresponds with the area of palpable concern and tenderness. There is a suggestion of mild skin thickening over the area of clinical concern. At this point, no additional mammographic views are needed, but ultrasound is indicated to further characterize the lesion. The differential diagnosis based on the mammogram alone includes infection, hematoma, breast carcinoma, and possibly inflammatory carcinoma (due to the focal skin thickening).

Ultrasound shows a poorly defined hypoechoic area with fluid tracking toward the skin surface and into the surrounding tissue planes. On physical exam, there was also erythema. At this point, the differential diagnosis becomes one of inflammatory carcinoma (localized) versus infection. The fact that there is a Hickman catheter buried in the tissue of the medial breast should be recognized on the mammogram, and on questioning, the patient had known septic emboli from an infected catheter. The ultrasound finding of tracking of fluid toward the skin surface is suggestive of an abscess that is heading toward spontaneous drainage through the skin. If there is evidence of an abscess collection, this area may be aspirated and sent for culture. Short-term follow-up and continued antibiotic therapy were recommended. The follow-up mammogram obtained 4 weeks later showed complete resolution.

Breast abscesses are most common in lactating women but also occur spontaneously or from seeding from another infected site, such as in this case. *Staphylococcus aureus* and streph bacteria are the most common agents. Clinically, there may be only cellulites or, as the case advances, an abscess may develop. Frank abscesses seen on ultrasound appear as mixed-echo masses with fluid debris levels, and even echogenic air may be seen. Treatment may include either percutaneous drainage with antibiotic lavage or open surgical drainage and excision.

Notes

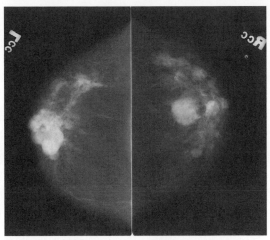

CCs

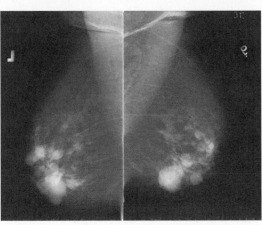

MLOs

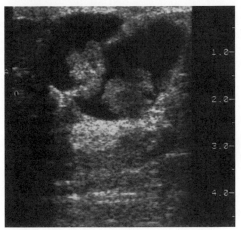

US

1. A 72-year-old woman presents with bilateral breast masses. Describe the mammographic findings.

2. Describe the ultrasound findings (similar for the multiple masses bilaterally).

3. Give a differential diagnosis for these bilateral masses.

4. What is the procedure of choice in this patient with bilateral breast masses?

Bilateral Papillary Carcinoma

1. There are bilateral masses with associated architectural distortion. Some of the masses appear to be slightly spiculated.

2. Ultrasound shows that there are bilateral intracystic masses.

3. The differential diagnosis includes multiple bilateral benign papillomas or multiple bilateral papillary carcinomas.

4. The appropriate procedure is somewhat controversial. Although core biopsy may establish the diagnosis of cancer, the core may also reveal atypia and complex sclerosing papillary lesions. In this case, bilateral excisional biopsy of the largest palpable masses was recommended, and bilateral invasive papillary carcinomas were found pathologically.

Reference

Wagner AE, Middleton LP, Whitman GJ: Intracystic papillary carcinoma of the breast with invasion, *Am J Roentgenol* 183(5):1516, 2004.

Cross-Reference

Ikeda, *Breast Imaging: THE REQUISITES*, pp 106–109.

Comment

Papillary carcinoma is more common in an older patient population and frequently presents as a solitary palpable mass or masses most often in the subareolar location. The masses are frequently round or macrolobulated, and as they become larger they often cause some architectural distortion or nipple retraction. Less common is the multiple bilateral presentation of papillary carcinoma, as in this unusual case. The patient had no symptoms of nipple discharge but was aware of growing masses in her breasts for many years. On ultrasound, these masses are often highly vascular and may have cystic areas; however, they may also appear as entirely solid masses.

Histologically, there are frequently areas of cystic change and hemorrhage. A distinction between intraductal and the invasive form may be difficult due to the large amount of chronic inflammation and stromal fibrosis that surrounds the mass. The prognosis of papillary carcinoma is excellent because the tumors tend to be slow growing. Lymph node metastases occur less commonly than in invasive ductal carcinomas, not otherwise specified.

Notes

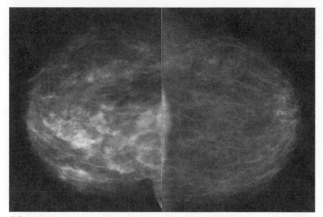

CCs 5 years later

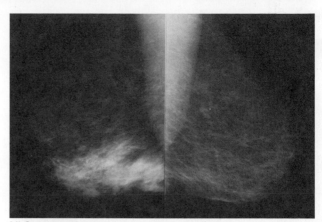

MLOs 5 years later

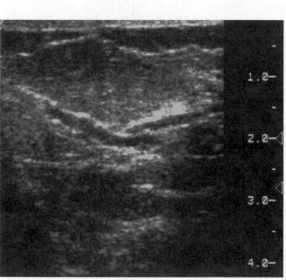

US of left breast

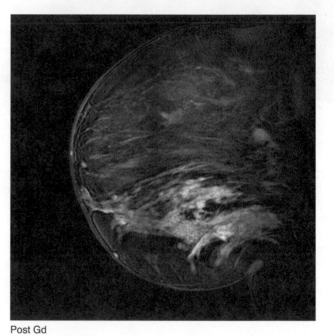

Post Gd

1. Describe the mammographic findings.
2. Describe the ultrasound findings.
3. Describe the MRI findings.
4. Biopsy reveals noncomedo DCIS. Name two subtypes of this form of DCIS.

Micropapillary Carcinoma

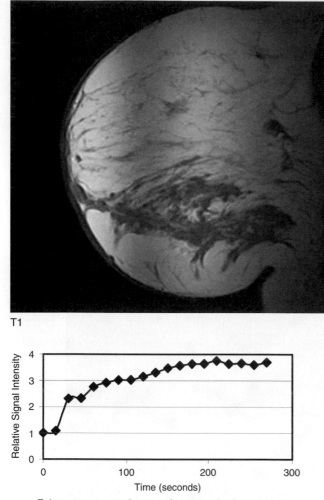

T1

Enhancement curve for area of segmental enhancement inferiorly on the left

1. There is a segmental focal asymmetry suggesting multiple dilated ducts mammographically.

2. Ultrasound shows dilated ducts that correspond to the mammographic abnormality. No masses are seen.

3. Multiple dilated ducts with a progressive regional enhancement were seen in the inferior breast in the area that corresponds to the ultrasound and mammographic findings.

4. Cribriform and micropapillary DCIS are noncomedo forms.

Reference

Bassett LW, Jackson VP, Jahan R, Fu YS, Gold RH: *Diagnosis of Diseases of the Breast*, Philadelphia, 1997, Saunders.

Cross-Reference

Ikeda, *Breast Imaging: THE REQUISITES*, p 82.

Comment

DCIS may be divided into comedo or noncomedo types or may be classified into high-, intermediate-, and low-grade forms. In this unusual case of extensive DCIS, biopsy revealed two noncomedo forms of DCIS: micropapillary and cribriform cell types. These histologic patterns tend to have a lower nuclear grade and slower growth rate compared to comedo carcinomas. The cribriform pattern refers to the multiple sieve-like spaces that form within the duct, histologically giving rise to the Latin term *cribrum* or sieve. The micropapillary form is characterized by proliferating cells that form projections or so-called "Roman arch" patterns within the dilated ductal structures and can present as a very extensive ductal dilatation with or without nipple discharge.

The imaging changes due to this type of cancer may be difficult to detect if no calcifications are present. In this case, mammographically there is a global asymmetry developing over an extended period of time as the segmentally dilated ducts become more evident in the inferior breast. Ultrasound reveals prominent ducts with thick echogenic walls, which is a nonspecific finding. On MRI, the areas of dilated ducts show very little enhancement and no intraductal masses are seen. Biopsy was recommended to differentiate between benign ductal ectasia and DCIS.

This case represented a very well-differentiated DCIS with a low nuclear grade and, hence, a very slow growth rate. The ducts became distended with a solid cellular proliferation, and because of the slow growth rate and small amount of neovascularity, there is very little enhancement seen on MRI. This patient had more than 10 cm of involvement of intraductal carcinoma. This is consistent with a very low nuclear grade and low mitotic activity of the cells.

Notes

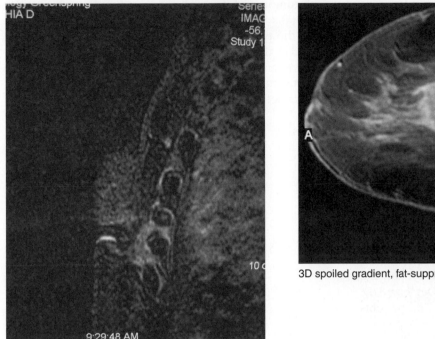

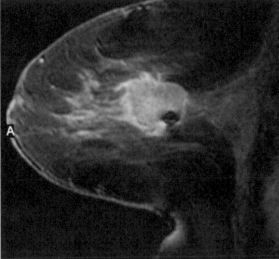

3D spoiled gradient, fat-suppressed post Gd

3D spoiled gradient, fat-suppressed post Gd

1. Describe the MRI findings in these two different patients.

2. Is there involvement of the pectoral muscle in either case?

3. Is there another radiologic modality that better depicts spread of malignancy to the chest wall?

4. Is it clinically important to assess whether there is chest wall involvement when reading breast MRI?

CASE 136

Chest Wall Involvement in MRI

1. Both patients have a suspicious enhancing mass in the posterior aspect of the breast.

2. There is enhancement of intercostal muscle in the first patient. There is tenting of the pectoralis in the second patient without definite malignant involvement.

3. MRI is the most accurate method of detecting chest wall involvement—better than mammography, ultrasound, and computed tomography.

4. It is important to assess and report enhancement of underlying muscle to allow the surgeon to better plan the excisional biopsy.

References

Morris EA, Schwartz LH, Drotman MB, Kim SJ, Tan LK, Liberman L, Abramson AF, Van Zee KJ, Dershaw DD: Evaluation of pectoralis major muscle in patients with posterior breast tumors on breast MR images: Early experience, *Radiology* 214(1):67–72, 2000.

Orel SG, Schnall MD: MR imaging of the breast for the detection, diagnosis, and staging of breast cancer, *Radiology* 220:13–30, 2001.

Cross-Reference

Ikeda, *Breast Imaging: THE REQUISITES*, p 217.

Comment

MRI is very useful in the evaluation of known breast cancer. It is used to evaluate the extent of disease and to check for additional masses in the same breast and in the opposite breast. MRI-detected unsuspected multifocal and multicentric ipsilateral cancer is reported to range from 16 to 37%. Occult synchronous contralateral cancer has been reported on MRI in 5–10% of cases, higher than that detected by mammography and physical exam.

MRI is also useful to determine the extent of disease beyond the breast by direct extension into the pectoralis muscle and into serratus muscle and intercostal muscles. The distinction between extension into pectoralis major and into underlying chest wall is important: Pectoralis extension alone does not affect staging, but chest wall involvement is designated as distant metastases.

In order to diagnose muscle involvement, look for enhancement of the muscle—more than the physiologic enhancement normally seen in nearby areas of muscle. The enhancement may be a diffuse involvement or may show enlargement of the muscle. Obliteration of the fat plane between the malignant mass and the pectoralis major muscle is not a definite indication of involvement with tumor, and it may be seen in tumors that abut the pectoralis but do not involve it.

In the two examples, the first patient has enhancing tumor in the intercostal muscle. In the second patient, there is an irregularly marginated mass with a biopsy defect. There is tenting of the muscle toward the mass but no definite evidence of malignant spread.

Notes

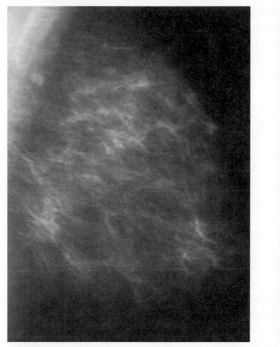

Right MLO

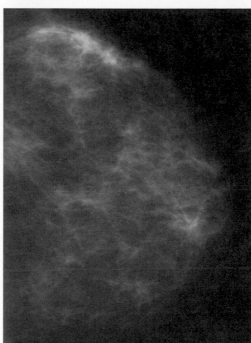

Right CC

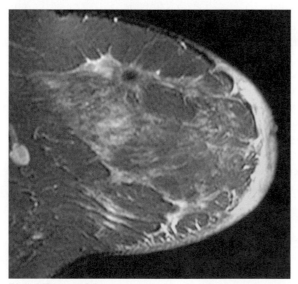

Right MRI post Gd

1. This patient presents with erythema and skin thickening in the anterior right breast. The mammogram was interpreted as normal at an outside location, and MRI was requested. What is in your differential diagnosis based on the clinical presentation?.

2. Describe the findings on the MR.

3. Does the MR help narrow the differential diagnosis?

4. What is the next step?

Inflammatory Cancer

1. The clinical findings suggest mastitis. The differential diagnosis includes inflammatory cancer.

2. There is a suspicious, irregular, enhancing mass in the upper right breast and marked skin thickening with enhancement. An enhancing node is seen at the chest wall.

3. The MRI appearance is consistent with inflammatory breast cancer.

4. Biopsy is needed. In this case, a skin biopsy showed adenocarcinoma.

References

Dershaw DD, Moore MP, Liberman L, Deutch BM: Inflammatory breast carcinoma: Mammographic findings, *Radiology* 190:831–834, 1994.

Gunhan-Bilgen I, Ustun EE, Memis A: Inflammatory breast carcinoma: Mammographic, ultrasonographic, clinical, and pathologic findings in 142 cases, *Radiology* 223(3):829–838, 2002.

Kushwaha AC, Whitman GJ, Stelling CB, Cristofanilli M, Buzdar AU: Primary inflammatory carcinoma of the breast: Retrospective review of mammographic findings, *Am J Roentgenol* 174(2):535–538, 2000.

Cross-Reference

Ikeda, *Breast Imaging: THE REQUISITES*, p 299.

Comment

This 40-year-old woman noted skin changes in her anterior right breast, with thickening and erythema of the skin. No mass was appreciated. She presented to her physician, who ordered a mammogram, which is shown. Because the mammogram was interpreted as normal, MRI was requested. The MRI shows marked thickening of the skin with enhancement, which corresponds to the pathologic finding of tumor in the dermis. There is also an enhancing mass in the upper outer quadrant of the breast, seen better on MRI than on the mammogram. Skin biopsy was performed and showed adenocarcinoma in the dermis extending to the deep dermis, with vascular invasion in the deep dermis.

Inflammatory breast cancer is so named because the breast can appear inflamed—red, swollen, and warm to the touch. This appearance is due to infiltration of breast cancer into the skin and lymphatics, causing edema and erythema of the skin. Edema gives a *peau d'orange*, or orange peel, appearance to the skin. It is usually recognized clinically, and its clinical appearance overlaps with that of mastitis or infection.

Skin changes in the breast are not exclusive to inflammatory breast cancer; they can also be seen after breast surgery and radiation therapy, mastitis, superior vena cava thrombosis, congestive heart failure, and lymphoma. Clinical history is important to eliminate these causes of breast erythema and edema.

With this clinical presentation, infection may be the most likely diagnosis. It is not unusual to try a course of antibiotics to determine if the erythema and skin thickening respond. If there is complete response of the clinical signs and symptoms to the course of antibiotics, biopsy may not be necessary.

Inflammatory breast cancer is rare, comprising 1–4% of all breast cancer. Any tissue type of cancer may cause inflammatory cancer, but invasive ductal carcinoma is the most common. In order to make the diagnosis of inflammatory cancer, there must be invasion of the dermal lymphatics. Mammographically, skin thickening and increased breast density and coarsening of stroma may be seen, although mammographic findings may be subtle, as in this patient. Masses and calcifications may be present but may be obscured by dense breasts, coarsened stroma, and overlying skin thickening. Lymphadenopathy is often seen (58%). The reported incidence of bilateral disease varies widely from 1 to 55%.

Ultrasound is a useful next imaging tool after mammography in evaluating skin changes. Skin thickening and masses may be seen, and the mass may be seen to involve the skin. Lymph nodes can also be assessed. MRI can be used if mammography and ultrasound are inconclusive.

It is important to recognize clinical signs of breast cancer that may present in the skin and to pursue additional evaluation with biopsy and/or additional imaging, even if the mammogram is normal.

Notes

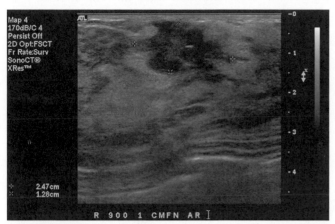

Initial presentation

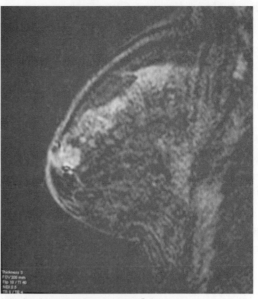

Initial subtraction image post Gd

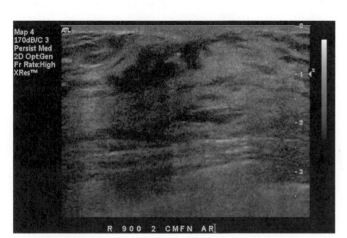

6 months later

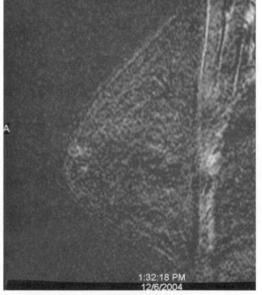

Subtraction image post Gd, 6 months later

1. This 27-year-old presents with a palpable mass in her right breast. Ultrasound was used for initial evaluation because of the patient's age. Describe the appearance of the palpable mass on the initial ultrasound.

2. The patient underwent a core biopsy and then adjuvant chemotherapy. What do you notice about the ultrasound of the mass between the initial presentation and 6 months later?

3. MRI of the breast was performed after the initial core biopsy. Describe the findings on MRI.

4. How do you explain the MRI appearance 6 months later?

Pre- and Post-Neoadjuvant Chemotherapy

1. There is a suspicious, very hypoechoic mass with angulated margins and duct extension.

2. The mass has decreased in size.

3. The subtraction view of the right breast shows an enhancing round mass with biopsy clip artifact. There is regional glandular enhancement in the upper right breast.

4. The mass is no longer seen on MRI after neoadjuvant chemotherapy. Biopsy clip artifact is seen. The glandular enhancement is no longer seen.

References

Balu-Maestro C, Chapellier C, Bleuse A, et al.: Imaging in evaluation of response to neoadjuvant breast cancer treatment benefits of MRI, *Breast Cancer Res Treat* 72:145–152, 2000.

Liberman L, Morris EA, Kim CM, Kaplan JB, Abramson AF, Menell JH, Van Zee KJ, Dershaw DD: MR imaging findings in the contralateral breast of women with recently diagnosed breast cancer, *Am J Roentgenol* 180:333–341, 2003.

Stavros AT, Thickman D, Rapp CL, Dennis MA, Parker SH, Sisney GA: Solid breast nodules: Use of sonography to distinguish between benign and malignant lesions, *Radiology* 196:123–134, 1995.

Cross-Reference

Ikeda, *Breast Imaging: THE REQUISITES*, p 214.

Comment

This 27-year-old presented with a palpable mass in June 2004. Ultrasound was the initial imaging study because of the patient's young age. (If a suspicious mass is seen on ultrasound, bilateral mammography is performed next, regardless of patient age.) Mammography is routinely the initial study in the setting of a palpable mass in women 30 years old or older.

In this patient, a suspicious mass was seen on ultrasound to correspond with the palpable finding. Her mammogram was normal, with dense tissue and no evidence of mass or microcalcifications. The next step in the evaluation includes biopsy of the suspicious mass.

A patient with breast cancer has a 1–3% increased risk of contralateral synchronous breast cancer at the time of detection of the primary cancer. Screening the breasts in the setting of a suspicious mass is most accurate using MRI as the screening tool.

This patient's right breast MRI, performed after needle core biopsy confirmed the diagnosis of infiltrating ductal carcinoma, showed only one suspicious enhancing mass and no evidence of additional masses. The left breast MRI was normal. This patient then received neoadjuvant chemotherapy—chemotherapy given prior to resection of the tumor. Follow-up imaging studies are performed after the chemotherapy to check the response of the tumor to the treatment. In this patient, the enhancing mass is no longer seen on MRI. There is a residual irregular mass on ultrasound 6 months later, which may represent fibrous tissue or residual malignancy. At surgery no residual malignancy was found.

Notes

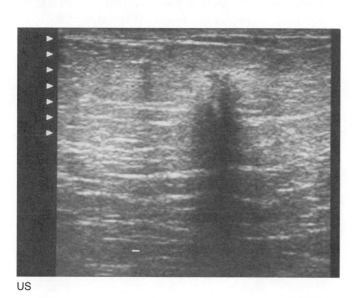

US

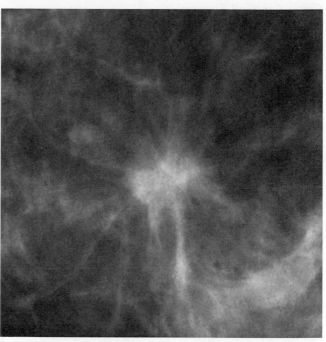

Spot mag

1. This 25-year-old medical student presented with an area of palpable concern in her right breast. Because of her age, an ultrasound was performed as the first workup. Describe the ultrasound findings. What additional imaging is recommended?

2. A mammogram was performed because of the highly suspicious ultrasound finding. Describe the findings and give a BI-RADS category.

3. On histology, granular esonophilic cytoplasm was present in bundles and cords with dense fibrous stroma. What, if any, further procedure is recommended?

4. What is the prognosis for this patient?

CASE 139

Granular Cell Tumor

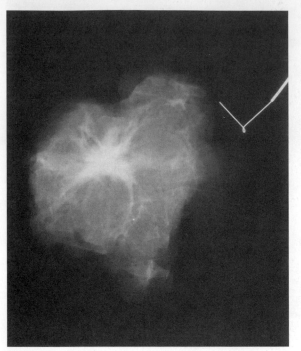

Specimen

1. A small, irregular hypoechoic mass with posterior acoustic shadowing was seen.

2. The mammogram shows a spiculated mass that corresponds to the area of palpable concern. BI-RADS category 4: suspicious, biopsy is recommended.

3. The histologic results are concerning; however, they are not indicative of invasive ductal carcinoma. These findings are due to a granular cell tumor. Excision is needed.

4. Most of these lesions are benign, and therefore the prognosis is excellent after a wide surgical excision.

Reference

Feder JM, Shaw de Paredes E, Hogge JP, Wilken JJ: Unusual breast lesions: Radiologic-pathologic correlation, *RadioGraphics* 19:11–26, 1999.

Cross-Reference

Ikeda, *Breast Imaging: THE REQUISITES*, p 91.

Comment

Granular cell tumors are unusual benign lesions that were initially thought to have a muscular origin but are now thought to derive from Schwann cells. They frequently occur in the tongue and other soft tissues of the body, and approximately 8% occur in the breast. They tend to occur at a younger age than breast cancer and occur more frequently in women than men.

The ultrasonographic, mammographic, and clinical presentation mimics breast cancer. The lesion usually presents as a painless, immobile, and firm mass that is often fixed to the pectoral fascia or chest wall and is spiculated mammographically. Microcalcifications are rare. On ultrasound, the lesion is irregular and cannot be differentiated from a category 5, invasive breast cancer. The frequent clinical picture of skin retraction or dimpling is also highly concerning for breast cancer. In this case, the very small lesion was quite palpable and was highly suspicious on mammographic and ultrasonographic imaging. A core biopsy was initially performed, and the diagnosis of a benign granular cell tumor was made. Most of these tumors should be cured by a wide local excision; however, rare malignant cases have been reported.

Notes

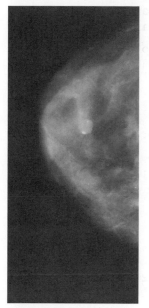

Displaced CC

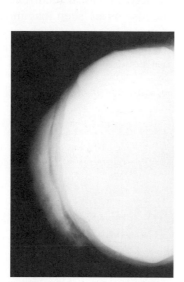

Implant CC

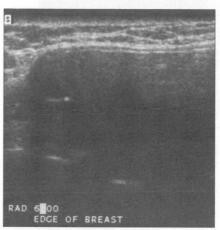

US of implant

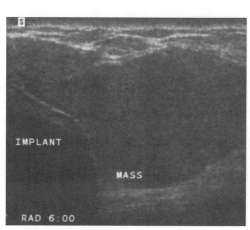

US mass

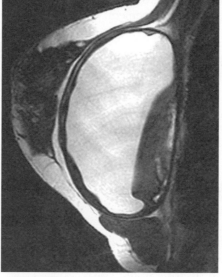

T1 sagital MR

1. This patient presents with a midline mass just below her right silicone implant. The mammography was not helpful because the mass was obscured by the overlying silicone implant. Describe the ultrasound and MRI findings.

2. What is the most likely differential diagnosis in this patient?

3. Could the mass be somehow associated with the fact that she has an implant?

4. What is the BI-RADS category and what, if any, procedure is recommended?

Desmoid

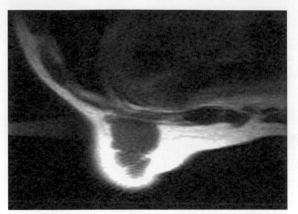

T1 axial MR inferior to implant

1. The ultrasound and MRI show a homogeneous large solid mass just inferior to the implant.

2. The most likely differential diagnosis is a giant fibroadenoma, extraabdominal desmoid, or some form of sarcoma.

3. Desmoids have been described growing in the surgical lines associated with implant placement.

4. This is given a BI-RADS category 4, and a core biopsy was recommended.

Reference

Feder JM, Shaw de Paredes E, Hogge JP, Wilken JJ: Unusual breast lesions: Radiologic-pathologic correlation, *RadioGraphics* 19:11–26, 1999.

Cross-Reference

Ikeda, *Breast Imaging: THE REQUISITES*, p 309.

Comment

This patient has an extraabdominal desmoid, which is an extremely rare benign infiltrating mass composed of a localized proliferation of mature fibroblast and collagen. Desmoids are more typically found in the abdominal wall. Extraabdominal desmoids usually present as firm, nontender, palpable masses that occasionally may be fixed to the pectoralis fascia or chest wall. They may be associated with dimpling, retraction, or edema and have clinical and imaging findings very similar to those of cancer. The masses may also occur in surgical lines, such as in this case, inferiorly along the surgical insertion site of the silicone implant.

Extraabdominal desmoids or fibromatosis of the breast may be associated with Gardner's syndrome. The diagnosis may be made by core biopsy, but since this benign lesion is locally aggressive, once the diagnosis is made, a wide excision is necessary. There is an approximately 20% local recurrence rate in the first 5 years. If the lesions are seen mammographically, they present as a mass, frequently with spiculation. On ultrasound, a hypoechoic solid mass with varying degrees of posterior acoustic shadowing has been described.

Notes

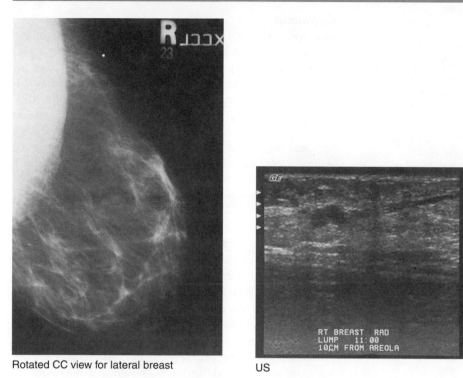

Rotated CC view for lateral breast　　　US

1. A 47-year-old woman presents with a palpable "cordlike" area in the axillary tail of the right breast. Describe the mammographic findings.

2. Describe the ultrasound findings.

3. What is the most likely diagnosis?

4. What is the clinical significance of this finding?

Mondor's Disease

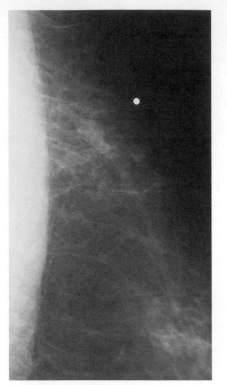

Cropped rotated CC

1. A tortuous "beaded" vessel is seen mammographically corresponding to the area of palpable concern.

2. Ultrasound revealed a dilated vessel with a filling defect and abrupt termination. No flow was seen on Doppler imaging.

3. This case is an example of Mondor's disease or superficial thrombophlebitis of the breast.

4. This disorder in uncommon but is usually iodiopathic, but may be associated with trauma. It is rarely associated with a breast malignancy.

Reference

Conant EF, Wilkes AN, Mendelson EB, Feig SA: Superficial thrombophlebitis of the breast (Mondor's disease): Mammographic findings, *Am J Roentgenol* 160:1201–1203, 1993.

Cross-Reference

Ikeda, *Breast Imaging: THE REQUISITES*, pp 305–306.

Comment

Mondor's disease, or superficial thrombophlebitis of the breast, most frequently presents with skin redness, pain, tenderness, and a palpable cord. There may also be associated skin dimpling or retraction, which may be concern for malignancy. The condition is usually idiopathic but may be associated with some sort of trauma to the breast, such as surgery, core biopsy, or excessive physical activity. It has also been described in cases of severe dehydration. The condition most frequently affects the thoracoepigastric and lateral thoracic veins. Rarely, this disorder is associated with a primary breast malignancy.

Mammographically, the thrombosed vein is a rope-like or beaded focal asymmetry, most often located in the upper outer quadrant or axillary tail of the breast. Sonographically, the superficial vein is often isoechoic or filled with low-level echoes due to clot. If imaged with Doppler imaging, there may be a flow void or abrupt cutoff of visible flow in the vessel. The condition usually resolves within 6 weeks with symptomatic treatment (i.e., hot compresses). The combination of the imaging and clinical findings should be adequate to make the diagnosis of this benign process. Biopsy is unnecessary, but the imaging should be carefully reviewed to exclude the rare associated malignancy.

Notes

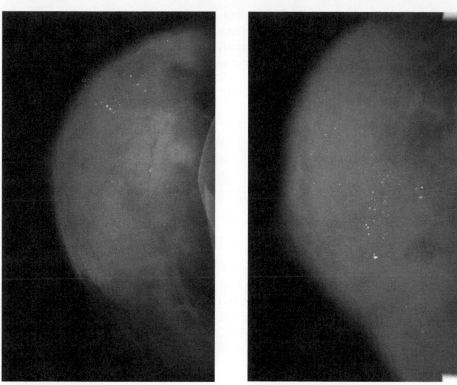

Left CC view cropped   Left MLO view cropped

1. How would you characterize the microcalcifications?

2. The patient has been lactating until very recently. Is this related?

3. Can you be sure the calcifications are benign?

4. If the calcifications are worrisome, does ultrasound play a role in the workup?

Lactational Calcifications

1. The calcifications are predominantly punctuate, with some amorphous forms and segmental distribution.

2. There is a relationship between lactation and developing calcifications.

3. No. While many of the calcifications have a benign punctate appearance, but some are indeterminate, amorphous, and slightly irregular shapes.

4. Ultrasound can be used to evaluate any related suspicious masses with associated calcifications.

References

Mercado CL, Koenigsberg TC, Hamele-Bena D, Smith SJ: Calcifications associated with lactational changes of the breast: Mammographic findings with histologic correlation, *Am J Roentgenol* 179:685–689, 2002.

Stucker DT, Ikcda DM, Hartman AR, George TI, Nowels KW, Birdwell SL, Goffinet D, Carlson RW: New bilateral microcalcifications at mammography in a postlactational woman: Case report, *Radiology* 217:247–250, 2000.

Cross-Reference

Ikeda, *Breast Imaging: THE REQUISITES*, p 287.

Comment

This 38-year-old patient with maternal history of breast cancer, who recently finished lactating, presented for a baseline mammogram. Microcalcifications are seen in both breasts, but are more numerous in the left. The calcifications are predominantly punctate, with some amorphous forms, and the distribution is segmental. The appearance is suspicious, BI-RADS 4.

Microcalcifications are most often the result of a benign condition, such as fibrocystic change, in which the calcium seen is in a tiny cyst or may be within the stroma. In ductal carcinoma *in situ*, the calcifications are in the ducts and represent necrosis of tumor cells. The appearance of the calcifications on mammography may be definitely benign or can be quite suspicious or indeterminate. In this patient, the calcifications are somewhat suspicious, so biopsy is recommended.

Calcifications may be seen in women who are lactating or have recently stopped. These calcifications may be related to inspissated secretions in benign ducts and also may be related to the involutional change occurring in the breast after lactation ceases. Of course, cancer may also occur in this population, and if the appearance of the calcifications are suspicious, biopsy is necessary.

In this patient, needle core biopsy was performed using the stereotactic approach because the ultrasound exam was normal. Histologic diagnosis of the calcifications was benign lactational change.

Notes

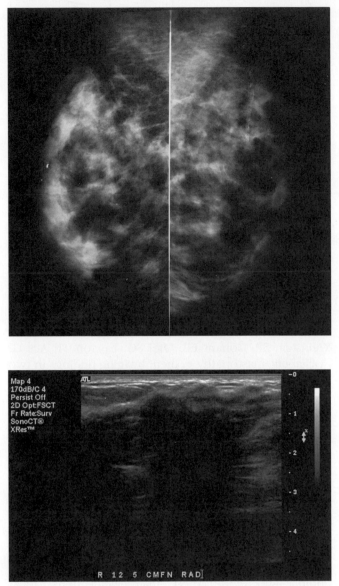

US

1. This patient has insulin-dependent diabetes with associated nephropathy. There is a palpable finding in the right breast at 12:00. What is in the differential diagnosis?

2. The mammogram shows a dense breast but no focal mass. Is this common in this condition?

3. Does ultrasound help in the differential diagnosis?

4. This patient has had previous ultrasound exams showing similar findings and has had multiple prior needle biopsies, all benign. Is there an alternative to core needle biopsy in this patient?

Diabetic Mastopathy

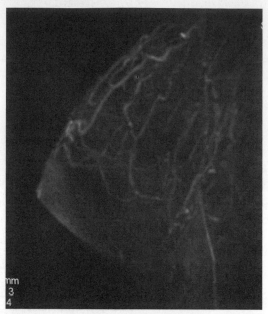

MR maximal image pixel projection (MIPP)

1. Diabetic mastopathy, malignancy, benign mass, and cyst.

2. Most patients with diabetic mastopathy have dense breasts with no focal finding to explain the palpable mass.

3. Ultrasound shows a hypoechoic, shadowing mass with indistinct margins. This ultrasound appearance is suspicious for malignancy.

4. Biopsy may be the best way to exclude malignancy and can be performed with needle core biopsy with ultrasound guidance in this patient. However, with known diabetic mastopathy, MRI can also be used to evaluate for suspicious enhancement.

References

Gabriel HA, Feng C, Mendelson EB, Benjamin S: Breast MRI for cancer detection in a patient with diabetic mastopathy, *Am J Roentgenol* 182:1081–1083, 2004.

Logan WW, Hoffman NY: Diabetic fibrous breast disease, *Radiology* 172:667–670, 1989.

Weinstein SP, Conant EF, Orel SG, Lawton TJ, Acs G: Diabetic mastopathy in men: Imaging findings in two patients, *Radiology* 219:797–799, 2001.

Cross-Reference

Ikeda, *Breast Imaging: THE REQUISITES*, pp 308–309.

Comment

Diabetic mastopathy is a condition that occurs in patients with long-standing insulin-dependent diabetes, typically young women but occasionally men. It may present with a firm palpable mass or bilateral firm masses on physical exam. The mammogram of diabetic mastopathy is very dense and there may be focal asymmetry, but there should be no mammographically suspicious findings—no evidence of microcalcifications, focal mass, or architectural distortion. Ultrasound features of diabetic mastopathy are similar to those in malignant masses: focal hypoechoic areas that have irregular margins and intense posterior shadowing.

In this patient, there is a new palpable finding in the right breast. She has already undergone several benign needle core biopsies in the past, with histology of dense fibrosis consistent with diabetic mastopathy. Mammogram shows dense breast tissue with no focal mass, and ultrasound shows hypoechoic area with posterior shadowing. The patient requested MRI to try to avoid additional biopsy.

On MRI, fibrosis should not show suspicious enhancement. The MRI of the right breast is shown, and no abnormal areas are seen. The patient was recommended to obtain routine follow-up.

Notes

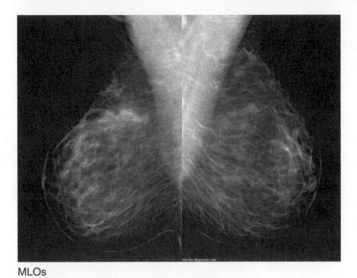

MLOs

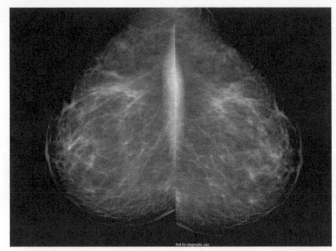

CC views

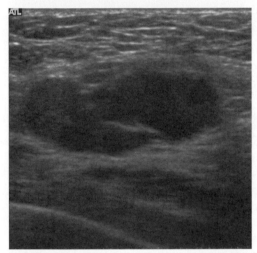

US left axillary node

1. This patient presents with a palpable mass in the left axilla. Are there any mammographic findings?

2. Describe the ultrasound findings from the left axillary ultrasound.

3. A FNA was performed of the left axillary mass yielding carcinoma, most likely from a breast primary. How often does breast cancer present as adenopathy with a negative mammogram?

4. What is the next imaging recommendation?

Axillary Node Presentation

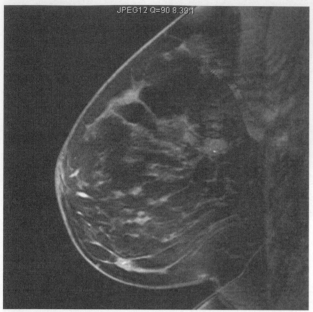

Left MRI pre Gd

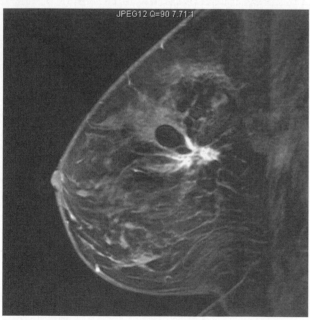

Post Gd

1. The mammogram is negative.

2. The ultrasound reveals an enlarged lymph node that corresponds to the palpable mass. The node appears abnormal, with a compressed or absent hilum and eccentric lobulated contours.

3. Breast cancer presenting as axillary adenopathy with a negative clinical breast exam and mammogram is very unusual, occurring in less that 1% of cases.

4. An MRI should be performed to look for a breast primary. In this case, the MRI demonstrates an avidly enhancing area of architectural distortion as well as an enhancing mass. The entire area spans approximately 4 cm and was shown on biopsy to be an invasive lobular carcinoma.

References

Morris EA, Schwartz LH, Dershaw DD, van Zee KJ, Abramson AF, Liberman L: MR imaging of the breast in patients with occult primary breast carcinoma, *Radiology* 205:437, 1997.

Orel SG, Weinstein SP, Schnall MD, Reynolds CA, Schuchter LM, Fraker DL, Solin LJ: Breast MR imaging in patients with axillary node metastases and unknown primary malignancy, *Radiology* 212: 543–549, 1999.

Cross-Reference

Ikeda, *Breast Imaging: THE REQUISITES*, p 213.

Comment

Breast cancer can present as isolated axillary metastases with no mammographic or clinical evidence of the primary cancer within the breast. Although this is a relatively rare presentation of breast cancer (less that 1%), MRI is particularly useful in detecting the otherwise occult breast primary. In two series of patients presenting with axillary metastases, MRI found the primary breast cancer in approximately 80% of cases, with the average size of the primary tumors ranging from 2 to 20 mm.

In the past, patients presenting with axillary metastases from breast cancer who had a negative mammogram and breast exam were treated with mastectomy. However, if an otherwise occult tumor is detected with MRI and the extent of disease established, the patient may be offered breast conservation therapy. Series have shown that there is no survival difference in this population between those who undergo mastectomy and those who have breast conservation with radiation.

In this case, the patient presented with a solitary left axillary node that on ultrasound appeared clearly abnormal. The node was enlarged and the central fatty hilum compressed, suggesting pathologic involvement. The mammogram was negative. The differential diagnosis at this point included a reactive lymph node, lymphoma, or metastatic tumor. A FNA yielded adenocarcinoma, most consistent with a breast primary. The MRI reveals the highly suspicious lesion in the posterior lateral breast that has avid enhancement and on biopsy yielded invasive lobular carcinoma.

Notes

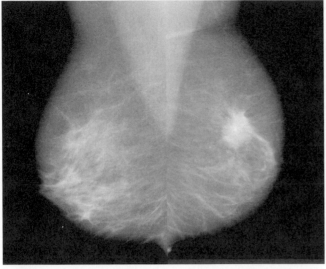

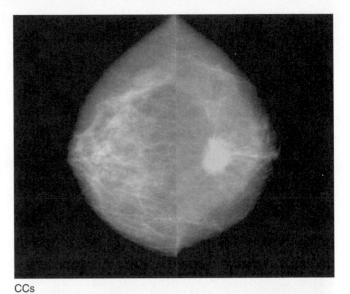

MLOs

CCs

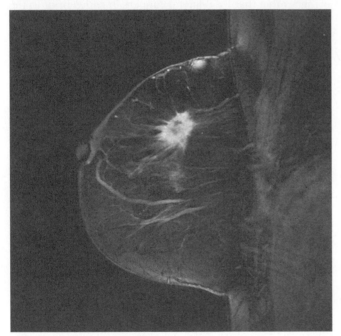

Right breast subtraction MR

Left breast

1. This 46-year-old patient presented with a palpable invasive ductal carcinoma in the right breast. The mammogram of the contralateral left breast was interpreted as negative. What is the likelihood that MRI screening of the contralateral breast will detect a synchronous cancer?

2. Describe the right breast MRI findings.

3. A 7-mm avidly enhancing mass was detected only on the postgadolinium images when the contralateral left breast was screened with MRI. Is this a suspicious finding?

4. What would be the next appropriate step to evaluate the left breast MRI finding?

Contralateral Screening on MRI

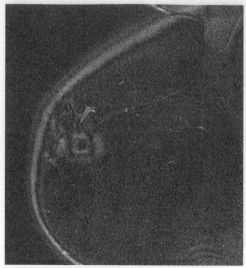

Left breast lateral needle

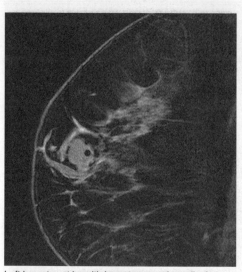

Left breast post bx with hematoma and needle tip

1. There is an approximately 4% to 10% synchronous cancer detection rate in the contralateral breast with MRI screening.

2. There is an avidly rim enhancing spiculated mass in the central right breast. This is the patient's known invasive ductal carcinoma.

3. Yes. The 7-mm mass in the right breast showed rapid, avid enhancement and then washout over time. This is a highly suspicious finding.

4. The small lesion in the left breast should be biopsied. A directed ultrasound may be able to locate the lesion so that ultrasound-guided core biopsy could be performed. Alternatively, the lesion could be biopsied under MRI guidance, as in this case.

References

Kriege M, et al., the Magnetic Resonance Imaging Screening Study Group: Efficacy of MRI and mammography for breast-cancer screening in women with a familial or genetic predisposition, *N Engl J Med* 351:427–437, 2004.

Lee SG, Orel SG, Woo IJ, Cruz-Jove E, Putt ME, Solin LJ, Czerniecki BJ, Schnall MD: MR imaging screening of the contralateral breast in patients with newly diagnosed breast cancer: Preliminary results, *Radiology* 226:773–778, 2003.

Cross-Reference

Ikeda, *Breast Imaging: THE REQUISITES*, pp 210–211.

Comment

Recent series have shown that MRI can detect otherwise occult contralateral cancers in patients diagnosed with a unilateral cancer in up to 10% of cases. This percentage is higher that that for bilateral cancers in series prior to the use of MRI. In longitudinal studies of patients diagnosed with a unilateral cancer, the incidence of contralateral cancers had been reported to be approximately 1% per year. The higher detection rate with MRI suggests that the contralateral cancers may be at least partially treated by systemic chemotherapy, which may delay or prevent their growth over time. Although the detection of contralateral cancers may impact survival, this has not been proven.

In this case, the right breast cancer was evident both clinically and mammographically, but the contralateral, left breast, 7-mm invasive ductal carcinoma was occult to conventional imaging. A directed ultrasound was performed to locate the left breast lesion but was unsuccessful. This patient underwent an MRI-guided core biopsy of the left breast lesion. Shown here are images obtained during the MRI core procedure. The needle was placed from the lateral aspect of the breast and the small mass was seen at the tip of the needle. Often by the time the core needle is placed, there is no longer contrast in the suspicious mass, as in this case. Fiducial markers on the skin, careful measurement of the depth from the skin surface to the lesion when contrast is evident, and identification of surrounding persistent glandular and ligamentous landmarks help confirm that the placement of the needle is correct. The images show the artifact of the needle shaft as it enters the lateral breast and the tip artifact more centrally at the lesion. Postbiopsy images revealing a hematoma at the biopsy site. A clip is placed to mark the biopsy site in case future excision is necessary.

Notes

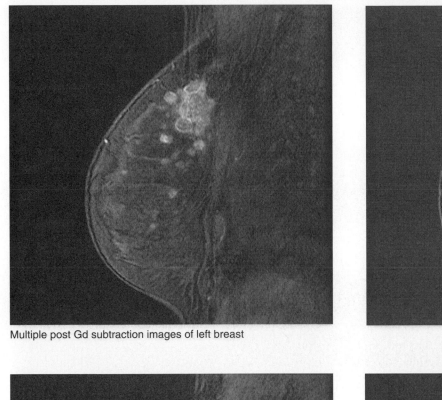
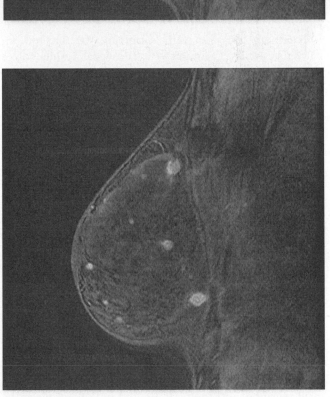

Multiple post Gd subtraction images of left breast

1. This patient presented with a palpable mass in the upper outer quadrant of the left breast that was also visible as a spiculated mass mammographically. The lesion was thought to be confined to the upper outer quadrant. What do the multiple MRIs demonstrate?

2. What is the definition of multifocal disease?

3. What is the definition of multicentric disease? Does this patient have multifocal or multicentric disease?

4. Why is accurate mapping of the disease extent important?

MRI Staging

1. There are multiple rim enhancing masses in the left breast consistent with extensive cancer.

2. Multifocal disease is cancer confined to one quadrant.

3. Multicentric disease is cancer in more that one quadrant. This patient has multicentric disease. The disease is seen both above and below the nipple axis and is both medial and lateral.

4. Accurate mapping of the extent of disease helps plan the appropriate surgical approach-breast conservation therapy (lumpectomy and radiation) or mastectomy.

References

Holland R, Veling SH, Mravunac M, Hendriks JH: Histologic multifocality of Tis, T1-2 breast carcinomas. Implications for clinical trials of breast-conserving surgery, *Cancer* 56(5):979–990, 1985.

Jacobson JA, Danforth DN, Cowan KH, d'Angelo T, Steinberg SM, Pierce L, Lippman ME, Lichter AS, Glatstein E, Okunieff P: Ten-year results of a comparison of conservation with mastectomy in the treatment of stage I and II breast cancer, *N Engl J Med* 332:907–911, 1995.

Orel SG, Schnall MD: MR imaging of the breast for the detection, diagnosis, and staging of breast cancer, *Radiology* 220:13–30, 2001.

Cross-Reference

Ikeda, *Breast Imaging: THE REQUISITES*, pp 213–214.

Comment

Among the major factors influencing the recurrence rate in patients who have had breast conservation is the extent of any remaining tumor in the breast after lumpectomy. Although adjuvant radiation therapy after lumpectomy is the clinical standard of care and has a major role in reducing recurrence rates, the local recurrence rates are reported to be as high as 19% at 10 years. The rates of recurrence in this population are higher in patients with extensive intraductal components, positive or close surgical margins, and multicentric and multifocal disease.

When serial sectioning of mastectomy specimens is done in patients with clinically suspected unifocal disease, up to 40% of patients have additional malignant foci in the breast. Certainly, if more extensive disease can be detected with MRI, and the disease is surgically removed by either an extended lumpectomy or mastectomy, the recurrence rates should decrease. However, long-term studies demonstrating the impact of this MRI staging on survival and recurrence rates are not available. This patient underwent a mastectomy that confirmed the presence of multicentric invasive ductal carcinoma.

Notes

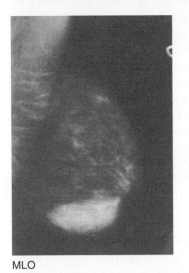

MLO

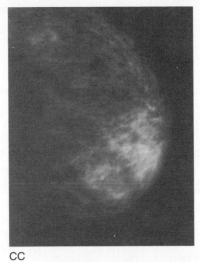

CC

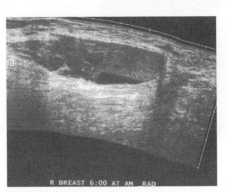

Rad US

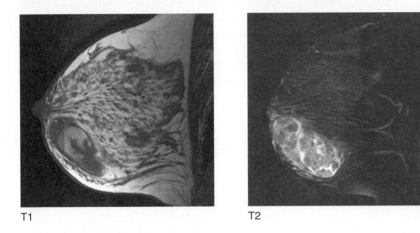

T1   T2

1. A 42-year-old woman presented for a screening mammogram. She was called back for additional imaging of the right breast. Describe the mammographic finding.

2. Describe the ultrasound finding.

3. An MRI was performed for further evaluation. Describe the findings on the multiple series presented.

4. What is the most likely diagnosis and BI-RADS category?

Hamartoma

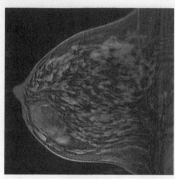

Post Gd

1. There is a large focal asymmetry in the inferior right breast that is of mixed density (appears to be partially fatty).

2. The ultrasound reveals that there is a hypoechoic solid mass with an eccentric cystic area. The mass has echogenic internal septations, and the appearance is most consistent with a benign process on ultrasound, such as a fibroadenoma. However, the mass did not have the typical appearance of a fibroadenoma on the mammogram due to the mixed density on the CC view.

3. MRI shows that the mass is fat containing (T1 image). In addition, the cystic component is seen, and there is a fluid level best seen on the T2 fat-suppressed image that is obtained at the edge of the lesion. The postgadelinium images show that the mass enhances, as does the surrounding breast tissue.

4. The findings are consistent with a benign hamartoma, BI-RADS category 2: benign.

Reference

Georgian-Smith D, Kricun B, McKee G, Yeh E, Rafferty EA, D'Alessandro HA, Kopans DB: The mammary hamartoma: Appreciation of additional imaging characteristics, *J Ultrasound Med* 23(10):1267–1273, 2004.

Cross-Reference

Ikeda, *Breast Imaging: THE REQUISITES*, p 120.

Comment

Hamartomas, or fibroadenolipomas, have a wide variety of appearances on mammography and ultrasound. Classically, the lesions have been described as well-encapsulated masses composed of glandular and fatty tissue found in varying proportions. Hamartomas are usually detected mammographically when the fat content is seen as areas of lucency, often with thin pseudocapsules where the hamartoma abuts the surrounding glandular tissue. However, more recently, it has been reported that hamartomas may have very little fat content and may present with imaging findings that mimic fibroadenomas. Ultrasound may show homogeneously hypoechoic masses with well-defined margins, making some hamartomas indistinguishable from fibroadenomas. Likewise, mammographically they may appear as dense masses with little or no fat apparent. When core biopsies are performed on these denser solid masses, the pathologic diagnosis of benign breast tissue or fibrocystic change may be indicative of a hamartoma.

In this case, the two mammographic images were confusing because the MLO suggested that there was a mass but the CC showed a mixed-density focal asymmetry. The ultrasound appearance of a large solid mass with fibrous septa and a large cystic space suggested a fibroadenoma or possibly a phyllodes tumor. The MRI confirmed the presence of fat in the lesions consistent with a hamartoma, and a biopsy was adverted.

Notes

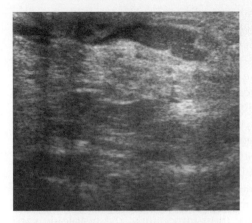
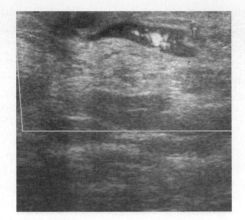

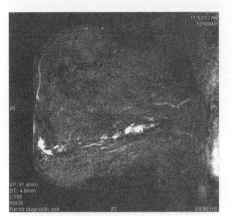

Subtraction MR image

1. This 53-year-old patient presents with spontaneous bloody nipple discharge. The mammogram was negative. Describe the ultrasound findings and give a differential diagnosis.

2. A MRI was recommended. Why might this additional test be helpful?

3. Describe the MRI findings and give a differential diagnosis.

4. How does the sensitivity of MRI in detecting DCIS compare with that of detecting invasive breast cancers?

MRI of DCIS

1. There is a prominent duct with what appears to be an intraductal mass in the subareolar location. This finding may be due to debris in the duct; however, the power Doppler image shows that the intraductal lesion is vascular and therefore not just due to debris. The differential diagnosis includes a benign papilloma as well as DCIS.

2. MRI has been shown to be very sensitive in detecting ductal abnormalities in patients with nipple discharge. Frequently, the extent of disease detected by MRI is greater than that detected by either mammography or ultrasound.

3. The subtraction MR image demonstrates not only the subareolar lesion that corresponds with the ultrasound finding but also suspicious ductal enhancement extending posteriorly in the breast.

4. MRI is less sensitive in detecting *in situ* cancers than it is in detecting invasive breast cancers.

References

Hwang SE, Kinkel K, Esserman LJ, Lu Y, Weidner N, Hylton NM: Resonance imaging in patients diagnosed with ductal carcinoma-in-situ: Value in the diagnosis of residual disease, occult invasion, and multicentricity, *Ann Surg Oncol* 10:381–388, 2003.

Orel SG, Schnall MD: MR imaging of the breast for the detection, diagnosis, staging of breast cancer, *Radiology* 220:13–30, 2001.

Cross-Reference

Ikeda, *Breast Imaging: THE REQUISITES*, pp 199, 236.

Comment

This patient with bloody nipple discharge was found to have extensive DCIS on excisional biopsy. There are quite a few ways in which this patient could have been evaluated (e.g., galactography), but in this case, with a negative mammogram, the breast imager chose ultrasound. An ultrasound of the periareolar area was performed and a single prominent duct with internal echogenic material was detected. This finding may be seen in benign ductal ectasia, but when power Doppler imaging was applied, the echogenic material was found to be highly vascular. Vascular intraductal lesions may be due to either benign papillary lesions or DCIS. At this point, a biopsy was recommended but a MRI was also recommended to further map out the extent of the disease.

The most common MRI findings in DCIS are ductal enhancement (as in this case) and clumped regional enhancement. Ductal enhancement patterns may also be seen in benign conditions such as multiple papillomas or ductal hyperplasia, but in this case an excisional biopsy of two sites was recommended; the anterior biopsy site was guided by ultrasound and the posterior site by MRI. The extent of DCIS found at the initial excisional biopsy required a mastectomy in this patient.

The sensitivity of MRI in detecting DCIS is quite variable in published series, from 40% to almost 100%. This sensitivity is significantly less than the MRI sensitivity in detecting invasive breast cancers. The wide variability in detecting DCIS is thought to be due to many factors, including the small numbers of cases in some of the series, the highly variable MRI techniques used in the small series, and, most importantly, the histologic variability (especially the variable degree of angiogenesis) seen in subtypes of DCIS. Improvement in imaging technique has been associated with improved detection, and a recent study showed that a balance between high temporal and spatial resolution is needed for improved DCIS detection. Investigators using a high temporal resolution protocol show a lower sensitivity in detecting DCIS than those using a high spatial resolution.

Notes

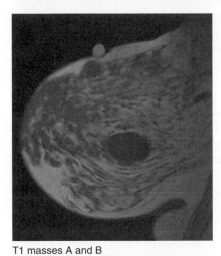

T1 masses A and B

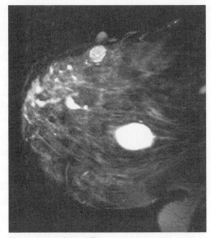

T2 masses A and B

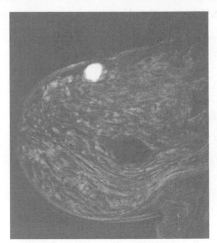

Subtraction image, mass A and B

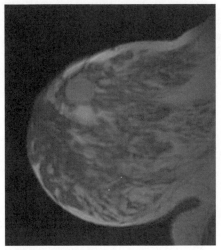

T1 mass C

T2 mass C

1. This high-risk patient had multiple masses on breast exam and was referred for a breast MRI. There are three large masses, A, B, and C (not all of the masses are visible on each MRI slice). Mass A is palpable. What type of marker is used to mark areas of palpable concern for breast MRI studies?

2. Based on the T1, T2, and post-contrast subtraction images, what is mass A most likely?

3. Based on the T1, T2, and subtraction images, what is mass B most likely?

4. Based on the T1, T2, and subtraction images, what is mass C most likely?

MRI—Multiple Masses

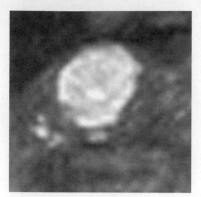

cropped T2 mag of mass A

1. A vitamin E capsule is used to mark areas of palpable concern because the fatty oil is well seen on the MRI sequences.

2. Mass A has low signal on T1, high signal on T2, showed progressive enhancement and has nonenhancing dark internal septations. This is consistent with a fibroadenoma.

3. Mass B has a low signal on T1, a high signal on T2, and shows no enhancement. This is consistent with a simple cyst.

4. A fluid debris level is seen in mass C. The signal is not as high on T2 as for the simple cyst or fibroadenoma due to the acellular debris in this complex cyst.

Reference

White Nunes L, Schnall MD, Orel SG: Update of breast MR imaging architectural interpretation model, *Radiology* 219:484–494, 2001.

Cross-Reference

Ikeda, *Breast Imaging: THE REQUISITES*, pp 199–203.

Comment

This patient has three dominant masses in the left breast. Mass A is superficially located and, since it is palpable, it is marked with a vitamin E capsule. Vitamin E or other oil-based capsules are used to mark areas of concern in the breast because they are highly visible on the MRI sequences.

Mass A is well circumscribed and has a high signal on T2-weighted imaging that may be due to either internal fluid or cellular material. The post-contrast images and the time enhancement curve reveal that the mass is solid with a progressive pattern—a pattern frequently associated with benign solid masses, not a cyst. Cysts may show very minimal rim enhancement but do not

enhance internally. The key to this case is the combination of the high signal on T2-weighted images, the progressive enhancement, and the nonenhancing dark internal septations best seen on the magnified post-contrast image that are almost pathognomonic of a fibroadenoma. The black internal septations represent the fibrous bands frequently seen in fibroadenomas. In younger premenopausal women, fibroadenomas may also show intense enhancement and even occasionally demonstrate a washout pattern of enhancement. When these more indeterminate features are seen on MRI, a recommendation for a biopsy may be necessary to exclude malignancy. In this case, however, the appearance is typical of a fibroadenoma and no further evaluation is needed.

Masses B and C are variations of benign cystic changes. On MRI, cysts generally show a low signal on T1-weighted images and a higher signal on T2-weighted images due to their internal fluid contents. Mass B is typical of a simple cyst with a fluid signal on T2-weighted imaging and no enhancement following contrast administration. Mass C is a complex cyst best demonstrated by the fluid debris level visible on all the image sequences.

Notes

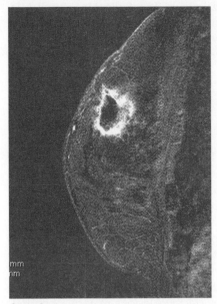

Case A

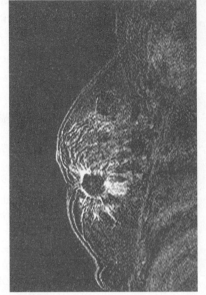

Case B

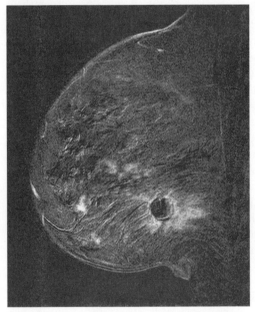

Case C

1. These subtraction MRIs from three different patients—A, B, and C—were all obtained approximately 3 weeks after the patients underwent lumpectomies. Why might MRI be helpful in cases like this?

2. Case A had a 1-cm invasive ductal carcinoma and negative surgical margins. Case B had an invasive ductal carcinoma and positive surgical margins. Case C had DCIS with positive margins. Describe the MRI findings in the three patients.

3. Do these findings suggest residual disease in any of the cases?

4. How specific is MRI in assessing for residual disease at the surgical margins in patients after lumpectomy?

MRI Assessment of Residual Disease

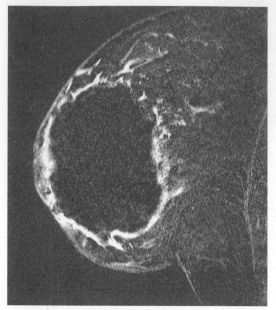

Case D, benign thin rim enhancement

1. MRI is useful in detecting multifocal and multicentric disease and may also suggest residual disease at the surgical margins in some cases.

2. Case A has a thick but even rim of enhancement around the surgical biopsy cavity. Case B has an enhancing mass at the posterior margin of the biopsy cavity. Case C has very suspicious enhancement in the tissue surrounding the surgical cavity as well as an area of linear enhancement anterior toward the nipple.

3. The findings in case A are nonspecific but, in view of the negative surgical margins, the enhancement is most likely due to benign granulation tissue. The enhancing mass at the posterior margin of case B is highly suspicious for residual disease. In case C, the enhancement around the biopsy cavity is suspicious for residual disease and the linear area anterior is suspicious for additional or multifocal DCIS. Case D (above) demonstrates benign, very thin rim enhancement around a large seroma.

4. MRI is moderately specific, but false positives may occur due to the avid enhancement of inflammatory tissue at the margin of the surgical bed when imaging is performed very early after surgery.

References

Frei KA, Kinkel K, Bonel HM, Lu Y, Esserman LJ, Hylton NM: MR imaging of the breast in patients with positive margins after lumpectomy. Influence of the time interval between lumpectomy and MR imaging. *Am J Roentgenol* 175:1577–1584, 2000.

Lee JM, Orel SG, Czerniecki BJ , Solin LJ, Schnall MD: MRI before reexcision surgery in patients with breast cancer. *Am J Roentgenol* 182:473–480, 2004.

Cross-Reference

Ikeda, *Breast Imaging: THE REQUISITES*, pp 236, 240.

Comment

MRI has been shown to be very accurate in estimating the extent of disease in patients with breast carcinoma. For patients considering breast conservation, it is known that complete removal of all tumor is associated with improved local control rates. Patients with close (<2 mm) or positive margins at initial excision routinely undergo re-excison if breast conservation is desired. If a lesion contained calcifications mammographically, postexcision mammographic imaging is necessary to assess for residual calcifications. However, mammography is often limited by the lack of compressibility of the breast, and postbiopsy changes and noncalcified or subtle calcified lesions may be obscured. Therefore, since MRI can depict both mammographically visible tumors and mammographically occult tumors, it is increasingly being used to guide treatment planning for women considering breast conservation.

A recent study evaluating MRI in patient with close or positive margins showed a sensitivity, specificity, and accuracy of 61.2%, 69.7%, and 64.6%, respectively. A thin, regular enhancing of 1 or 2 mm around the seroma cavity was considered normal (see case D), and any focal areas of nodular or mass-like enhancement were considered suspicious for residual disease. Unfortunately, early postoperative MRI assessment of surgical margins is limited by granulation tissue that forms around the margin of the surgical site. This inflammatory tissue may avidly enhance and cause false-positive interpretations for residual disease and even false negatives when intense rim enhancement obscures small focal enhancing areas of residual tumor. Optimizing the timing between surgery and MRI is important so that both false positives and false negatives are minimized. A recent study suggested that waiting approximately 4 weeks allows decreases in the enhancement due to inflammation and does not significantly delay any additional surgery.

The thick but regular rim enhancement in case A is a somewhat nonspecific finding, but in combination with known histologically negative margins and no evidence of multifocal or centric disease, no further surgery is necessary. Case B demonstrates a focal nodular area of suspicious enhancement that on re-excision represented residual invasive disease. Case C had MRI-detected residual disease at multiple surgical margins as well as DCIS detected away from the surgical bed that was biopsied under MRI guidance. The patient underwent mastectomy and had multifocal DCIS.

Notes